# A PRESCRIPTION TO KILL

Also by Thomas W. Giffin

*Cube 6*

# A PRESCRIPTION
## TO KILL

A NOVEL

Thomas W. Griffin

W
Watson Press
Seattle

Copyright to come

*To Griffin and Paige*

THERE'S BEEN A HORRIBLE ACCIDENT. A truck driver is trapped in the cab of his burning vehicle. Police, firemen, and EMT personnel are at the scene, but it's clear that the truck driver will burn to death before he can be freed from his truck. He's screaming, he's in terrible agony, and he knows that he's going to die. He begs a policeman to shoot him rather than let him burn. Legalities aside, which prevails: individual autonomy and freedom of choice, or the view that human life is precious and not for society to devalue?

A LAW LEGALIZING PHYSICIAN-ASSISTED suicide was passed in Oregon in 1997. Affirmed by the United States Supreme Court in 2006, it remains the only such law in the country. Since it came into effect, legalized assisted suicides have been responsible for approximately 0.1% of the deaths in that state.

# Prologue

IT STARTED WITH a little twitch. It wasn't much, just the faintest of movements, and he barely noticed it. But it was followed by a lingering tremor in his left hand. He shook it out and tried to ignore the sensation. Then it went away, and he thought nothing more of it. He got on with his day as if nothing had happened.

He awoke at 7:30 just like he did every morning, no alarm needed. He had his own internal alarm and it never failed. He showered, shaved, brushed his teeth, dressed, ate a light breakfast, and then, as was his habit, he scanned *The Wall Street Journal*.

He read an interesting article about politics, the upcoming election, and the future of health care reform. It led him to make a few quick stock trades. He wasn't exactly a day trader, but he did like to play the market, especially the health care stocks; and when it came to health care stocks, he won more than he lost, quite a bit more. But as he clicked on the "execute" icon to sell five hundred shares of Hospital Corporation of North America, the twitch came back again. His finger moved of its own accord. He watched it for a moment and then stopped it by force of will. The finger stilled, and although there was no tremor, he couldn't help but wonder, what was *that* all about?

He worked at his computer until 10:30 and then took his daily mid-morning walk to the Pony Espresso coffee shop. He sat at his usual table by the window and ordered a double tall nonfat cappuccino. He was enjoying the view when it happened a third time: His finger twitched. It tapped the table, disconnecting from the rest of his body as if typing some secret message all on its own. He watched its autonomous movement for a few seconds while the beginnings of a headache formed somewhere behind his eyes. Then he slapped it still by covering his left hand with his right.

The twitching stopped. He removed his covering right hand. The finger remained quiet. He made a fist. He flexed his fingers and worked them back and forth. When nothing else happened, he opened his *Journal* and read something about a Medicare fraud investigation in Florida. The article amused him. He knew a thing or two about Medicare fraud, and he smiled at the article's conclusions.

A waitress brought his cappuccino over to his table. She put his drink down in front of him and then asked him something, some kind of a question. He just stared at her, tilting his head to the side, trying to understand the words. They sounded wrong.

"Isth ythin els Ican ofo u?"

He wrinkled his forehead and then rubbed the wrinkles away with his fingers. He felt confused. What was happening?

She stood waiting for a response.

He squinched his eyes shut. His headache exploded. He pressed his hands to his temples. His eyes popped and opened wide. His pupils dilated. He blinked a few times, arched his neck, and then fired a stream of vomit all over his table, splashing it onto the waitress in front of him.

She jumped back and screamed a startled, clipped scream. His eyes rolled back in his head. People at the next table stood to get out of the way. Everyone looked in his direction.

His left hand started to flop wildly around like a dying fish. He knocked his cappuccino over into his lap. His water spilled. Glassware crashed. He attempted to stand, but his left knee buckled. He fell forward on his face. His leg shook as he slid down to the floor, pulling the tablecloth and everything on it down with him.

His entire body went into spasms. Someone screamed something, the cry sounding like "Cal lado tor!" He bit down hard on his tongue. Saliva foamed. His mouth filled with blood. And that's all he could remember.

# Chapter 1

OCEAN CITY, OREGON, was a quiet little town, or so it seemed when Dr. Carrie Williams first arrived. Its singular claim to fame was that Lewis and Clark had spent the winter there in 1805, making it the oldest settlement west of the Rocky Mountains. Its only hospital, the Sisters of Mercy Medical Center, was built by the Catholic Church for a growing population that never came. Always overstaffed, underoccupied, and filled with charity cases, it was on the brink of bankruptcy when it was bought and rescued by the Hospital Corporation of North America.

Carrie Williams was a chief medical resident on loan there from the University of Washington. She'd been sent to Ocean City for a four-month clinical rotation in community medicine. She was tall, a little over six feet, and could be strikingly beautiful when she wanted to be. Her hair was black, her eyes were brown, and her skin was a creamy mocha.

She'd just finished a prostate exam on an old logger named Furman Moseley and was sitting at the seventh floor nurse's station writing orders in his hospital chart when an elegant gentleman approached the other end of the counter. He asked the ward clerk if he could speak with Dr. Williams. Carrie turned when she heard her name. She made eye contact. "I'm Dr. Williams," she said. "May I help you?"

"I hope so." He was tall and tanned, had a touch of gray in his hair, and wore an expensive-looking lightly pinstriped charcoal-colored suit. His shoes were polished to a bright shine. He could have been anywhere between forty-five and sixty-five years old, and he looked very fit. "I'm Dr. Bennett; I don't believe we've met." He extended his hand. "I'm here to talk to you about a patient of mine, Stewart Wolf. I'm his private physician. I understand that he's been assigned to your inpatient service."

Carrie shook his hand. She noticed his clothes, his shoes, and his manner. He wasn't the usual small-town doctor. She was intrigued, maybe even a little charmed. "Stewart Wolf. ..." She thought for a moment. "That's right. He's one of mine."

"Can we talk?" he asked.

"Sure." She put down the hospital chart she held in her hand.

Bennett nodded toward the end of the hall. "I wondered if we could speak in private. It's something very important involving Mr. Wolf's care."

Now captivated by this new face of Ocean City medicine, Carrie led him to the family consultation room at the end of the hall. The space had been designed to be warm and comforting, a private place for patients and their families to meet with their doctors. Carrie didn't like the space; she thought the room felt much like Ocean City itself: insulated from the outside world.

Bennett took a seat on a couch. Carrie pulled up a chair. "We can talk here," she said. "No one will bother us. How can I help you?"

"I'm sorry to trouble you," Bennett said. "I remember what

your work is like. I did my residency at Hopkins, and there were never enough hours in the day to get things done. The last thing I needed was to have some private doc interrupting my routine." He shifted a bit on the couch. "As I said, I came here to talk with you about Stewart Wolf. I've been his doctor for a number of years. We've been through a lot together. And now, as you know, he's developed a brain tumor."

"A glioblastoma multiforme," she said.

"That's right. Pathologically it's a grade four. It's incurable."

"I agree. I saw his path report this morning. There's no question about the diagnosis."

"Okay, then. I see that you understand, so I'll get right to the point." He leaned slightly forward. His face expressed concern. "This is one of the worst cancers anyone can get. The average survival is only nine months. Stew was diagnosed last February; he's already had seven. Statistically, he has only two months left to live. But practically speaking, he has less than that. He's had the predictable severe headaches and episodes of projectile vomiting, and we've been able to control his symptoms for the most part with medication. His quality of life up until a few days ago has been generally good. But unfortunately that's all changed now."

"I know," Carrie said. She called up the image of Wolf's hospital chart in her mind. "He was admitted for treatment of a hemorrhagic stroke, if I'm not mistaken."

"Not exactly," Bennett said. "Actually, I think he bled into his tumor. At least that's what the MRI looks like, but that's neither here nor there." He paused for a second. "See, I didn't admit him for treatment in the conventional sense. His tumor's far beyond that." He paused again. "Two weeks ago, Janet—that's his wife—noticed a dramatic change in Stew's mental status. It was subtle at first, but then it accelerated. He started forgetting things—initially little things, but later bigger things, things like who he was, where he was, what he was doing, that sort of thing. He lost orientation as to time, place, and person, and since then he's had a rapid deterioration of his cognitive abilities.

"We put him on Decadron to take some of the pressure off of his brain, and he improved for a little while, but now he's back on his downhill course. He refused treatment with radiation. He said he didn't want any part of that. The same thing with chemotherapy. He knows he's going to die. Yesterday he became totally confused and started babbling on and on about all sorts of things, strange things, things that were very disturbing to his wife. He became quite agitated, and then he had a seizure. I had to sedate him to prevent him from hurting himself. Janet couldn't handle him anymore, so I admitted him to the hospital."

"But you said not for treatment?"

"No, not for treatment." Bennett reached into the inside breast pocket of his coat and pulled out a folded piece of paper. He unfolded it and then handed it to Carrie. "It's a living will," he said. "Stew told me a long time ago that he wouldn't want to live this way. He made his wishes quite clear, both to me and to his wife."

Carrie looked at the paper. She studied it. "This is a legal document?"

"It's a copy of the original," he said. "But it's notarized, and I recognize the handwriting to be his. It's legal, and it conforms to the dictates of Oregon's assisted-suicide law. I had my lawyer check it out before I came over here just to be sure. You can never be too careful with this kind of thing."

*Assisted suicide?* Carrie didn't know what to feel or say. "I've never done anything like this before." She avoided looking at his face, staring at the paper without really looking at it.

Bennett put his hand on her arm. "We all have to have a first time," he said. "It's just another part of medicine, a very important part. It's a shame that it doesn't get more coverage in medical schools."

"I'm from Washington." Carrie continued to stare at the paper. "It's not legal there. It's not legal anywhere other than in Oregon, at least not in this country."

Bennett sighed, "No, it's not. Places like your state, Washington, even have laws prohibiting it, so they do it there illegally, but they still do it. We're just allowed to be a little more honest about it down here."

Carrie's eyes left the paper and searched the room. She fingered the papers, thinking about her Hippocratic oath, an oath to preserve life; about her mother, she'd died an untimely death, languishing for a month in a coma; about Stewart Wolf, who didn't *want* to go on living in his condition. "I don't know ..."

"Maybe this will help," Bennett said. "Stew was my friend. He was a proud man, a strong-willed man, but there's little of that man left. And what does remain lives on in agony. Already he can't communicate effectively. And that's exactly why he told his wife and me, long ago, what he expected us to do if this happened to him. Have you had a chance to meet him yet, to examine him?"

"I've seen him," Carrie said. "I did his intake exam earlier today. He wasn't able to talk. Like you said, you have him pretty heavily sedated. She looked down at her shoes. "Do you really need me to do this? You can't find somebody else or do it yourself?"

"It takes two signatures. You're his resident, his inpatient doctor; it's your responsibility.

"The law is very specific; there are elaborate safeguards. Patients must be adults, they have to be mentally competent at the time they make their requests, and they have to make them twice, in writing, separated by at least a fifteen-day interval. Two persons not related to the dying person have to serve as witnesses. Stew's witnessed requests are attached to his living will." He showed Carrie the two witnessed and dated requests. "Then two independent physicians have to certify that the patient has six months or less to live. In my opinion, Stew has at most only six weeks, maybe only six days."

"But he isn't truly suffering," Carrie said. "He isn't in pain."

"Not now, but you should've seen him before he was medicated. His headaches were unbearable and unrelenting. They were driving him insane. Besides, there's no requirement for unbearable suffering in the law, and pain has nothing to do with it. Only one patient in the entire history of Oregon law has requested an assisted suicide for fear of intractable pain. It's more about dignity, that and the ability to control the circumstances of one's death."

"I'd like to discuss this with his wife," Carrie said. "I want to hear what she has to say firsthand. See how supportive she is of all this."

"Of course," he said. "I'd expect nothing less. Everyone's told me how conscientious you are, the university's resident of the year and all that. I wanted you to meet Stew's wife, too, and I brought her along. She's actually waiting for us downstairs in the hospital chapel." Bennett reached inside his coat to retrieve another document from his pocket. "I'll leave this with you," he said. He exchanged it for the living will. "It's a statement of medical prognosis. I've already signed it; you'll need to put your signature right below mine." He showed her the place to sign. "It details Stew's medical condition and says that under the best of circumstances he only has a few months left to live. If you're comfortable with this process after you've talked with his wife, sign it here and put it in his chart behind the copy of his living will."

Carrie looked away from the paper and out the window. The world outside was gray and foggy. Drizzle had coalesced on the glass, warping the view. It was a world without perspective. The outlines of trees and buildings were indistinct. Clouds hung low and ragged in what pilots call an indefinite ceiling, a condition that sometimes makes it difficult to maintain spatial orientation. No doubt that was how the world appeared to Stewart Wolf—to the extent he was aware of anything anymore.

Carrie turned back to Dr. Bennett. "When do you need this?"

"I don't want to push you," he said, "But for Stew's sake it would be best if we could get this done today. This whole thing's been very hard for Janet, Mrs. Wolf. I'd like to get it over with tonight so that Stew's at peace and she can get on with her life."

A few seconds passed, and then Carrie asked, "How do we do it? I mean, how is it done?"

"Morphine. We attach a morphine drip to his IV. Stew signed a durable power of attorney in the event circumstances such as these should arise. That document is also attached to his living will. He'll just drift off."

Carrie again looked down at the document. She waited quite a while before looking back at Bennett. "I'll go downstairs and talk to Mrs. Wolf," she said, "but no promises. I'll have to feel right about this. I just don't know. I'll let you know my decision later."

"Sure," Bennett said. "That's all anyone can ask." And with that said, they both stood up and left the room.

:   :   :

Carrie stopped by to see her patient on her way down to the chapel. His room was cold, too cold; she adjusted the thermostat.

Then she stood at the side of his bed for a while, simply looking at him.

The bed rails were down, and she raised them for his protection. He had an IV in his arm and a catheter in his bladder, and he was wearing a diaper. He was confined to the shell of his body. He would never get any better. He would never be whole again. This was no way to live.

She hesitated, and then on impulse she reached over the bed rail and gently shook his shoulder. Wolf moaned in response. She gently shook him again. This time he made no sound at all. He remained heavily sedated.

She whispered something into his ear. His eyelid twitched, but nothing else. She closed her eyes, searching for inspiration—or at least guidance. She received none. She slowly opened them again.

Wolf's hair was mussed, and Carrie smoothed a few errant strands away from his forehead with her fingers. His respirations were soft and steady.

"What are you thinking?" she whispered.

His thoughts were locked up inside his head.

Then she softly touched his cheek, took a few steps back, and turned to leave for the chapel.

:    :    :

The hospital chapel was small and dark, and the first thing that Carrie noticed was the smell, a smell of dust and old candle wax laced with just a trace of incense, nothing at all like the rest of the hospital. It looked and felt like what it was: a holdover, a relic from the hospital's original owners, the Catholic Church. It had seen little use since the Hospital Corporation of North America purchased it. It existed in its own separate building adjacent to the lobby, and it was attached only through a small side door.

Carrie had entered the building through the connecting door, and it took a moment for her eyes to adjust to the darkened room. The chapel walls were white, the beams supporting an arched gothic ceiling were dark brown, and there were three stained glass windows on either side of the sanctuary. The grimy windows depicted scenes from the Old and New Testaments, and they hadn't been cleaned in years. Like Ocean City itself, the chapel seemed to be suffering from a kind of gentle, benign neglect.

The main door to the chapel was located at one end, and there was an altar holding a large Bible, a cross, and several unlit candles at the other. Six sets of church pews were lined up on either side of a central aisle. Mrs. Wolf was dressed in a conservative dark suit and was sitting in the second pew on the left. Bennett was sitting beside her. The two of them looked up in her direction as she approached.

Bennett stood and said in a soft voice, "Janet, this is Dr. Williams."

"Do we really have to do this?" Mrs. Wolf asked.

"I'm afraid so," he answered. "I'll leave you two alone. I'll wait just outside." Bennett put his hand on top of hers, smiled a kind smile, and then pulled it away. He stood up and walked out through the door in the back. Janet Wolf followed him with her eyes.

Carrie waited for Bennett to leave and then said, "Mrs. Wolf?" She looked up into Carrie's face. Carrie could see that she'd been crying.

"Please," Janet Wolf indicated, motioning for Carrie to sit next to her and sliding over to make more room in the pew. "This is very difficult. I wish we didn't have to do this. It's hard for me to know where to start."

Carrie sat. "I understand. I don't mean to pressure you."

"Oh, I know. This is difficult for both of us." She folded her hands across her lap, and then after a few moments of silence she said, "What am I supposed to say? How am I supposed to ask you to help my husband die?" She began to cry again as she shook her head. "He's been my life for twenty-three years."

Carrie let her cry for a moment. "Dr. Bennett explained the situation to me. Just tell me what you feel, what you think he would've wanted if he could tell me himself. I need to know what he was like. I need to know his state of mind. It's my duty to carry out his wishes, but I need to know that his wishes haven't changed since he wrote his living will."

"I'll try," she said as she wiped her eyes with the back of her hand. "See, Stewart was, is, a strong man. Unlike me, he's never been afraid of anything. He's never been afraid to die." She looked up at Carrie as if seeking judgment.

"Just look at me," she said. "I'm scared to death." She held out her hand in front of her and watched it shake; then she lowered it and looked back into her lap. She sighed. "This is so difficult. Stew always said that he wouldn't want to linger. That's why he had our lawyer draw up that living will. It's very specific; that's just like him." She smiled a momentary smile as if recalling some distant memory. The tears started to run down her cheeks again. "It's just so awful. What else can I say?" She squeezed her eyes shut and silently started to sob.

Carrie reached over and touched her on her shoulder. "Do you have any children?"

"No, no children." She looked up at the altar.

"Any other relatives?"

"No," she sniffled. "There's just us. No one else. There's never been anyone else."

Carrie studied her for a moment. "I wish this were easier. I know that ... well ..." She searched for words. "Is there anything else that you'd like to tell me?"

The room was silent. The air was heavy. Carrie felt the weight of the sanctuary. Then through her sobs she said, "He was in such pain! It almost killed me to see him suffer like that. And now he's so helpless. He's ... he's ... ." Janet shook her head. She squeezed away her tears, slowly regaining her composure. "I never thought this would happen." She looked up into Carrie's eyes. "But now that it has, I want to do what my husband asked."

Carrie gently patted her on the shoulder. "I understand. We don't need to go any further with this. We'll honor your husband's wishes."

From behind them, Dr. Bennett cleared his throat, alerting them to his presence.

"Do you have a pen?" Carrie asked him.

"Certainly."

Carrie removed from her coat pocket the folded paper he'd given her. She signed it in the proper spot and then handed it back to him.

"Thank you, Dr. Williams." He took the document. "I'll see that it gets into the hospital chart." Then he added, "The only other thing I need from you at the moment is to order the morphine drip. I have to get back to the office to see a couple of patients. I'll come back and check on it later."

Carrie nodded, suddenly feeling exhausted. "It'll be done," she said.

With that, Bennett thanked her again, took Janet Wolf's arm, and left the chapel.

:　:　:

Carrie sat alone in the chapel. Filtered light streamed in through the dirty stained glass windows and surrounded her with a spider web of dark colors and shadows. She looked up at a grimy Moses threatening to break the stone tablets that he held high in the air over his head. The faint smells of incense, candle wax, and religious ceremonies long since past suddenly seemed oppressive. She listened for the choir but instead heard only an echo of Mrs. Wolf's words: *How do I ask you to help my husband die?* She needed to clear her head. If she still smoked, she would have needed a cigarette. Instead she needed some air.

She slid out of the pew, walked outside through the main chapel doors, and stood for a while in the cleansing Ocean City mist. Water droplets condensed on her cheeks. She wiped them off.

She took out her cell phone and called Tim Hixon, one of her old mentors in Seattle. Somehow she got immediately through to him. As soon as she heard his voice, she simply unloaded on the man. And like the angel he was, he listened patiently to her plight.

In measured tones, Hixon said he understood her predicament and that he wasn't sure exactly how Oregon law worked. He worried about the distinction between assisted suicide, which is permitted, and euthanasia, which is not. In view of the power of attorney, he assumed that the request for active assisted suicide was lawful, but just to be safe, he suggested that she write the morphine order for pain relief and sedation, not for suicide assistance. She could then let the drug do its work under the "double effect" principle.

"Ordering meds to end a life can be risky," he said, "but there's absolutely no risk in administering a drug for pain relief. And if as a side effect it shortens a patient's life, well ... it's safer for everyone to do it that way. That's how we do it in Washington, and that's probably how most physicians do it in Oregon in spite of their 'death with dignity' law. That's why their statistics for physician-assisted suicide seem so low."

"Thank you so much," Carrie said. "Thanks for listening, the advice, and everything. You don't know how much it means."

"I know you're facing a difficult decision," Hixon said. "It's one that we all have had to face at some time or other. But I also know you, Carrie. I absolutely trust that you'll do whatever's best for your patient. You always do. Trust in yourself and your judgment. You're one of our best. And let me know how it turns out."

"I'll do that," she promised, and then she said goodbye.

: : :

Stewart Wolf stared at the ceiling, looking at nothing. He lay suspended in a drug-induced state somewhere between sleep and wakefulness, aware and yet at the same time not aware of the world of the hospital to which he now belonged.

His medications were delivered intravenously, and it had been almost an hour since they'd added morphine to the concoction of drugs flowing into his veins. As per Carrie's orders, the flow rate had been initially set at a sub-lethal level. Prior to that, she had given Wolf a stimulant to wake him up so that they could talk about his medical condition and his living will. The stimulant had worked remarkably well—so well, in fact, that she and Wolf had talked about many things before the morphine finally took effect. Most important, Wolf had told her in his own words that he no longer wished to live. As the stimulant had worn off, though, his conversation had ranged off in various directions, ultimately degenerating into this state of semiconsciousness. Now his breathing was soft, his bed rails had been raised for his protection, and only the constant beeping of his heart monitor kept him anchored to the reality of the physical world.

Carrie checked on him one last time. She quietly approached the side of his bed and gently touched his cheek, asking softly, once again, if he could hear her.

He didn't respond.

She turned up the rate on the intravenous flow pump. Morphine concentrated in the tissues of his brain. He was floating away. She watched for a while and then left the room. He floated for hours more. Finally his heart rate slowed. His brain forgot to tell him to breathe. He depleted his stores of oxygen. His arms and legs twitched a few times. His body stilled. He blinked once. The computers monitoring his medical condition noticed a change in his physiological status. And then they sounded the alarm.

:   :   :

Carrie was catnapping in the residents' on-call room when the alarm went off and the speakers blared, "CODE BLUE, SEVENTH FLOOR, CODE BLUE, SEVENTH FLOOR, CODE BLUE, ROOM 721." Nurses rushed to the room with their crash cart, interns ran up the stairs to respond to the cardiac-arrest code, and Carrie Williams was jolted awake from her few moments of exhausted sleep. It had been a tough day—five admissions and a case of steroid psychosis—and she'd had little sleep the night before. And then on top of everything else, there was Stewart Wolf. Her eyelids were still etched by the rapid eye movements of her dreams.

Carrie stumbled out of bed a little disoriented, turned on the lights, and looked at the clock on her bedside stand. It read 3:14 PM. She tried to clear her head. Her pager started to chime. She reached for her knee-length white lab coat and pulled it on over her wrinkled green scrub suit. She checked the pager attached to her coat pocket, and it confirmed the location of the code.

"What the hell?"

Then she grabbed her stethoscope off the bedside stand, draped it around her neck, and hurried out of the room.

The code was well under way by the time she arrived. Wolf was lying in his bed on his back. Joe Unis, an intern, was sitting astride his body on his knees, pumping his, heart while Candy Peterson, a nurse, squeezed air into his lungs with an Ambu Bag. Wolf had been stripped of his sheets and bed covers, and his hospital gown had been opened, exposing his chest. A resuscitation mask connected to the tube extending from his mouth covered most of his face, but Carrie could still clearly see his vacant eyes—eyes that stared beyond the ceiling.

Someone had placed a wooden board under his back to facilitate the CPR effort. A system of plastic IV bags hung from a pole above an IV flow pump. It fed clear fluids into his veins through a snakelike section of IV tubing. Patty Forsman, another intern, was in the process of injecting 1,000 milliliters of bicarbonate solution into the tubing just below the flow pump. She'd already injected epinephrine. Carrie's job was to evaluate the progress of the resuscitation effort.

"How long?" Carrie asked.

"Twelve minutes since the computer alert," said a second nurse standing at the foot of the bed. Her name was Tina. She was holding Wolf's open hospital chart in her hand.

"Why the computer alert? The alarm should have been turned off. That's standard procedure with a DNR order."

"A DNR?" The nurse gave Carrie a puzzled look. "A do-not-resuscitate order?"

"Paddles!" Unis ordered. He hopped off the bed, rubbed the two defibrillator paddles together in their conducting gel, and then placed them firmly against Wolf's chest. "Clear!" He squeezed the red trigger on the paddle handle. Wolf's chest heaved, and then he fell back onto the bed. The cardiac monitor remained flatlined. It was their third attempt at electrical cardio stimulation.

"Nothing," Unis said.

Candy Peterson said, "I think he's gone."

The second nurse looked away from her patient and started to thumb through his chart. "He has an advanced brain cancer," she said as she flipped through the pages, "But we don't have a DNR order." She looked up at Carrie. "What do you want us to do?"

Carrie stared back at her in shock. "What do you mean, no DNR? I wrote that order myself."

The nurse again checked the order sheet. "Well, it's not here." She shook her head; then she held up the chart for Carrie to see.

"What?" Carrie was stunned. The chart was turned to the correct page, but the no-code order was gone. "But I wrote the order. It should be in there. Something must've happened to it."

Unis climbed back onto the bed and restarted the external cardiac massage. Candy restarted respiration with the Ambu Bag. One of Wolf's ribs snapped as Unis compressed his chest.

Carrie focused back on her patient. She moved to the bedside. She took a penlight out of her pocket and flashed it first in his left eye and then in his right. There was no light reflex. Both pupils remained fixed and dilated. "Stop pumping for a minute," she said. Unis and Candy both stopped their resuscitation efforts. The cardiac monitor remained quiet. "There's nothing there."

"It's been that way since I got here," Unis replied.

"Twelve minutes?" she again asked the nurse.

"Fourteen now."

Carrie rechecked the monitor. There was no evidence of cardiac activity. "Then that's it," she said. "It's over."

Candy removed the resuscitation mask from her patient's face. Unis climbed off his chest.

Carrie looked at Wolf's lifeless body for a moment. Then she spoke to the people around her. "Can anyone tell me what just happened here?" She looked around the room. "Anyone?"

The group was silent for a moment, and then Tina, the nurse

with the chart, answered, "I don't know. He seemed to be fine when we checked on him an hour or so ago. He's been sleeping peacefully. His vitals were all in the green, and then all of a sudden the alarm sounded."

"That's not what I mean," Carrie said. She again looked around the room. "Why are we doing this? Why are we coding a terminal patient?"

The nurse hesitated before she answered, "His heart stopped. We don't have an order for a DNR." She looked around at the others in the room for support. Nobody else said a thing.

Carrie said, "Come on. This isn't right. This wasn't supposed to happen." She looked back at her patient. A tube was protruding from his mouth. "This was supposed to be an easy death. He was supposed to just drift away."

The silence in the room was total. Nobody moved. All eyes were on Carrie.

"What? What's the matter? There's a copy of his living will and a statement of prognosis in his chart."

More silence. Then after a few awkward moments, the second nurse said, "We have your order for morphine, but there's no living will, no statement of prognosis." She again thumbed through the chart. "And there's nothing about turning the morphine up to a lethal level. There's nothing like that at all."

Carrie's mouth suddenly went dry. "May I see that?" The nurse handed her the chart. Carrie carefully went through it page by page. The documents were not where they were supposed to be. She thumbed through it again. She felt a shiver. Then she looked up as someone new entered the room.

He was a short, balding man in his mid-50s wearing a brown tweed sport coat, khaki pants and loafers. His tie didn't quite go with his coat. A loop of stethoscope tubing was hanging from his coat pocket. He stepped quickly across the room and was taking Wolf's wrist when Carrie stopped him.

"Who are you, and what are you doing in here?"

"I'm feeling for a pulse." The man looked up at her with gentle eyes. "With cardiac monitors and such, I know that it really isn't necessary, but it's an old habit." His eyes moved to her identification badge. "You're Carrie Williams, I see. I've heard good things about you."

With a growing sense of unreality and dread, Carrie asked him once more: "And who are you?"

"Oh, I'm Bill Bennett, Mr. Wolf's private physician."

# Chapter 2

SEATTLE, WASHINGTON, is supposed to be one of America's most livable cities. Tell that to Jon Kirk, a thirty-something-year-old, kick-ass, do-anything-for-a-story type of investigative reporter for the *Seattle Times*. He was weaving his way through heavy traffic on Madison Avenue, honking his horn at a delivery truck that had just cut him off while he was talking on his cell phone with Chris Collins, his city desk editor. According to the American Automobile Association, Seattle has the fourth-worst traffic in the nation; only Los Angeles, San Francisco, and Washington, D.C., are worse.

Collins was arguing with Jon about a story. "If the lawyers say no, then the answer's no! I don't care how good the story is; they have the final say. Always have; end of conversation. There's nothing left to talk about."

"Oh, come on," Jon said. "It wasn't a definitive no. It was just a wishy-washy lawyerly kind of a no, a qualified no. That's all. It's certainly no reason to gut the story."

Jon waited for an answer. The silence from Collins was deafening. Jon shrugged and kept driving.

Jon was in a hurry. He'd just had a major story published using information that his live-in girlfriend, Karen Able, had told him in confidence. Karen was a cop, a homicide detective with the Seattle Police Department, a job that hadn't always mixed well with his. He'd promised to meet her at six o'clock to discuss the indiscretion before their dinner date at the 1200 Bistro, and he was running late.

"Listen," Jon said, "what if I delete some of the more indelicate details, some of the 'how to' stuff? Would that mollify the lawyers?"

"It goes beyond that," Collins said, "and you know it. The legal team's concern is that people might act on some of the information in the article. We could be liable for their deaths."

Jon zipped around a school bus before it could extend its paddle and tie up traffic in both directions. Then he increased his speed and slid toward a break in the traffic. "The lawyers are just trying to protect their backsides. They teach it in law school, self-preservation 101."

A short, blond woman in an age-appropriate Mercedes darted out in front of him, turning onto Twenty-third Street. He braked hard, swerved to the left to miss her, and then accelerated again. He laid on his horn. Her personalized license plate read MARGI. She extended her middle finger.

Jon's story was about one of Seattle's leading citizens, Edwin McRory. He'd been slowly dying from liver failure, could no longer drink alcohol, had been too old for a liver transplant, and had recently arranged for a one-way trip to Switzerland to end his life with a physician-assisted suicide. Both assisted suicide (in which a lethal drug prescribed by a physician is administered by a patient) and voluntary euthanasia (in which a doctor or someone else administers a lethal medication) had been legal in that country since 1942. McRory had left a note explaining what he was going to do and why he was going to do it, and among other things in the note he'd lamented Washington State's lack of an assisted-suicide law. The note had come to light during a police investigation related to an issue with McRory's insurance policy.

Karen had seen the note and had briefly mentioned it to Jon. Jon then obtained a copy from one of his other sources at the SPD and published his article. During his research he'd learned that the Swiss handled most of their assisted suicides through "right to die" charities and that *Dignitas*, the best known of the group, had dedicated itself mainly to non-Swiss citizens. By doing so *Dignitas* had created, in effect, a government-sanctioned but underground assisted-suicide tourist trade. Jon had just completed a fabulous follow-up feature on the subject for the newspaper's Sunday edition. And he wasn't about to let Collins spike it, lawyers or no.

"Come on, Jon," Collins said. "Make the changes the lawyers suggest. We've saved a spot for a page-one lead-in. The bones of your story are great, but as written it's practically an instruction manual for suicide. Our governor's going to push for a new law here in Washington next year anyway. It's near the top of her agenda. You can see the problem from the owner's point of view. Bend a little bit, will you?"

"I've already bent a lot. There's a suicide-tourism industry springing up in Europe, and our readers deserve to know how it works, especially with the potential for a new law here."

A black Hummer zipped by, crowding Jon away from the centerline.

"Your angle's great," Collins said, "but we can't print it the way you've written it. If you'll just …"

"Then I'll take it to *The Weekly*," Jon interrupted. "I'll do it;

you know I will."

"You, a Pulitzer Prize-winning reporter, writing for *The Weekly*? That's a laugh. Surely you can come up with something better than that."

"Try me," Jon said simply as he stopped at the Martin Luther King stoplight. The light turned green, and Jon stepped hard on the accelerator.

Collins took a deep breath and let it out. "I think we need a little time out here. Listen, I'll talk to the legal department again and see what I can do. We ought to be able to reach some sort of acceptable agreement."

Jon turned left onto McGilvra Street. His house was half a block away, and he was running out of time. "OK, Chris, talk to the lawyers. Get them to negotiate. But just remember, I'm not moving on this; my position's not negotiable." He pulled up to the curb in front of his house. "Call me back when you get an answer." He flipped his phone shut with a snap.

Jon was self-aware enough to realize that he'd always had difficulty with authority. But there was authority, and there was stupidity. One he could respect; the other, never. But now he was home, and he had to put all of that out of his mind. He had more pressing problems. Karen would be waiting for him somewhere inside.

:     :     :

Jon cautiously opened his front door and walked into his house. Leon, his basset hound, greeted him at the front door. Karen was in the bedroom dressing for dinner.

"Hi, Karen," he said in a cheerful voice. He heard her moving around, but she didn't answer. He knew that she'd heard him. *Uh-oh.*

Jon quietly walked up the stairs into the bedroom. "You're not still mad at me, are you?" he said to her back. Her red hair swept across her bare shoulders as she walked into the bathroom to apply a touch of makeup. She was wearing black bikini panties and a matching bra.

"I said I was sorry. I thought we'd called a truce." He slipped into the bathroom behind her, wrapped his arms around the tight muscles of her waist, and gently pulled her close to him. He watched her reflection in the bathroom mirror as she tried to suppress a smile.

He nuzzled her neck. "Well, say *something*."

"Something." She leaned closer to the mirror to finish her eye makeup.

He persisted as he again gently tugged her in to him to make body contact. "Come on, Karen; tell me you forgive me. I'm sorry; I really am. It was all a big mistake. It'll never happen again." Theirs was a relationship made in heaven, almost.

Karen spun around. "You can be a real ass, you know that? You deliberately took the information I told you in confidence and published it without my permission. You got one of your slimy friends in the SPD to give you a copy of McRory's suicide note, and then you published it. Why would you use me like that?" She pushed him away from her.

"Please, Karen, I really am sorry." Jon's eyes were apologetic. "It's just that once I talked with the McRory family and found out how passionate they were about the assisted-suicide cause, how much they wanted his views publicized, well, I guess I got carried away. It was always my intention to consult you. I would've, but ... ."

Karen took a step back and punched him hard in the shoulder. "Ouch!" She knew how to throw a punch; she used her shoulder, not her arm. Her soft beauty disguised a sinewy strength. She was one of those athletic types who worked out in the police department's gym, and she was a whiz with the speed bag.

"Don't you ever think about the consequences of your actions?" she asked. "How do you think you made me feel? Now everyone in the department thinks that I leaked that story to you."

"But you didn't leak it." Jon rubbed his shoulder.

"I might as well have. I told you about the suicide note. You wouldn't have known about it if I hadn't told you. Why can't you follow the rules like everybody else?"

"Karen, I ... ."

"Oh, shut up." She stepped forward, pulled him into her and kissed him softly on the lips.

Jon kissed her back. "I'm forgiven?"

"You've been given a reprieve, at least for the moment." She playfully bit his lower lip a little harder than she needed to. "Now go away and get dressed. I changed our reservations. We're going to the Ewe Club. Chef Tom is expecting us. This little episode is going to cost you big time." She pushed him away, turned back around to the mirror, and finished her eyes, then brushed on a little lipstick.

Chef Tom was a master chef, the best in the city and the most expensive. Jon wondered how much credit he had left on his Visa card.

His cell phone rang. The LCD read, "Chris Collins." He tried to ignore it; it rang again. "Shit." He reluctantly answered, "Hi, Chris. Could I call you back? I'm a little busy right now." He was looking at Karen in the mirror.

"I would, but something just came up. Go to your computer. Check out the AP wire, keyword 'Carrie Williams.' There's been a murder in Ocean City, Oregon. A resident physician from the University of Washington is accused of killing one of her patients."

"Uh-huh." Jon walked slowly toward his computer. "That's interesting. Well, as I said, I'm a little busy right now. And until we can resolve the other issue … ."

"It's taken care of. The lawyers backed off. We'll publish your suicide tourism piece as is, but we need you to do this one first."

"Ah, why this one first?"

"Number one, because you're going to want to do it first, and number two, because we'll get scooped if you don't get on it right away. The resident in question claims that she's been tricked into what she thought was an assisted suicide. She says it's only now that she realizes it was a murder. She claims an impostor posing as her patient's family doctor got her to do it. She says she was duped."

Jon paused and then asked, "This is a joke, right?"

"No, no joke. Her patient's dead. She killed him. Obviously this story ties in with your Switzerland work *and* the McRory article. Like I said, I'll keep the lawyers off your back. You have my word on that. Just get down there and get to work. Right now."

"I have your word on the lawyers?"

"That's what I said."

"All right, then." Jon looked at his watch, "I'll, uh … ." He glanced up and saw that Karen had been listening to his side of the conversation. She'd wiggled into a little black cocktail dress and was giving him a stern warning glare as she turned her back for him to zip it.

"Jon? Jon?" It was Collins, still on the line.

"I'll get there by first light." Before Collins could answer, Jon flipped the phone shut and reached over to zip Karen's zipper.

Karen turned to face him. A smile replaced the glare as she smoothed her dress over her taut body. She touched him lightly on his sore shoulder, nuzzled in closer, and said, "Good call."

# Chapter 3

THE INQUEST STARTED after evening rounds, precisely at seven. Dr. David Bolam, the chief of staff, sat at the center of a long, narrow mahogany table. He was dressed in a navy blazer, gray slacks, and a muted blue tie. He was flanked by six members from the hospital staff and board, three to his left and three to his right, and he faced Carrie sitting in a single chair on the opposite side of the table. A large paneled nook on the wall behind him originally held a Madonna, a holdover from the hospital's previous owners; now it contained only empty shadows. There was a faint smell of furniture polish in the air. With its dark wood paneling and blood-red deep-pile carpeting, the hospital's boardroom was designed to impart a feeling of *gravitas*.

After formally greeting Carrie and bringing the inquest to order, Bolam addressed the assembled group. "Each of you was given a copy of Stewart Wolf's medical history along with Dr. Bennett's account of events. You also have Dr. Williams' response. I assume you've all had a chance to read it." There was some shuffling of papers, but nobody spoke. Bolam then addressed

Carrie. "Dr. Williams, do you have any comments on the report?" She shook her head. "Good, then we can proceed.

"As you know, we're here to investigate the circumstances surrounding the death of Stewart Wolf." He paused for a moment. His tone was measured. "Please tell us in your own words exactly what happened, and feel free to take as much time as you need. Tell us everything, and be as complete as you can. With these conflicting reports," he gestured toward the printed handouts, "we need to understand exactly how this unfortunate set of circumstances came to pass." Roger Bower, a board member and the hospital's legal counsel, wrote something down on the legal-sized pad sitting in front of him.

There was a preliminary discussion among the members of the group. Even after the conversation abated, Carrie didn't answer right away. She searched Bolam's eyes. She scanned the faces on the opposite side of the table. The room stilled. She took her time, she cleared her throat, she swallowed, and then, finally, she began.

"Before I came to Ocean City ... ." She started with a history of her medical background, telling them about her residency training, her experience, and the university contract that brought her to their community. Her inquisitors followed her monologue with polite attention. She spent several minutes discussing her patient, Stewart Wolf, his diagnosis, and his initial medical work-up. She told them about the treatment of glioblastoma multiforme and how the survival rate, even with the best treatment, was essentially zero. She mentioned her interactions with other members of the hospital's house staff and the role that Dr. Unis and the other interns played in her patient's care.

Finally Alexandra Morse, the hospital's CEO, interrupted her presentation. "We know all of that," she curtly said. "Let's skip the preliminaries and move ahead, shall we? We're wasting time here." Morse was in her mid-thirties, a little young for a chief hospital administrator, and was dressed in a tailored Chanel navy blue suit. Her skirt was cut short, and along with her three-inch heels it was designed to flatter her long legs. "Tell us about your conversations with Wolf." She wanted to know if they'd discussed the particulars of physician-assisted suicide.

Roger Bower held up his hand. "Hold on, Alex. We agreed to give Dr. Williams as much time as she requires. We have legal obligations."

"That's all right," Carrie answered. She turned to Morse. "I tried to talk with him about it, and I thought that he understood. He was sick of living in his state of dependency, and everything that he said was consistent with his living will." She went on to tell her and the group about his problems with mentation and continence, about his lack of control over his other bodily functions, and about his expected quality of life.

Then she took a deep breath and told them about the impostor. She described in detail how he looked, how he talked, how he seduced her with his story, and about the missing living will and statement of prognosis.

"Did you ever ask him to show you his credentials?" It was Joe Drozda, a staff physician.

She admitted that she hadn't. "But he knew everything about Mr. Wolf's case. He was really good. No one would have guessed that he wasn't who he said he was."

"Then he might have actually been an M.D."

"It's possible."

She went on to tell them about her discussions with the woman who claimed to be Mrs. Wolf, and she told them about writing the order for morphine, about the cardiac arrest code, and about her ensuing confrontation with Dr. Bennett.

She continued answering their questions for at least another hour, and after she finished she felt exhausted but confident.

Bolam looked down at his notepad; he'd been writing notes during their discussion. After reading for a moment he said, "Does anyone have anything else that they'd like to ask?" He looked first to his left and then to his right. No one spoke. Next he addressed Carrie. "Is there anything else that you'd like to add?" She started to say something but then changed her mind and shook her head no. "Then I assume that your testimony's complete," he continued.

"At least for now," she answered. "But if you require any additional information in the future …"

Bolam looked up. Their eyes locked. They stared at each other for a moment. He clenched his lips and shook his head back and forth. "Dr. Williams," he said, "I don't know how to put this any other way. I'm disappointed in you. You tell an incredible story, and I think it best if …"

"Just a minute!" she interrupted. "What do you mean by incredible? It's the truth, and with a little more time I'm sure I can find people to back me up. There were other people up on the ward, people who must have seen the impostor. I'd even be willing to take a lie detector test."

Bolam cleared his throat, cutting her off. "That may be very helpful, but before we get into all of that, there are some things that we need to take care of here." His voice was firm and his eyes were cold.

He continued, "To begin with, I want to warn you that you

should seek legal counsel."

Carrie looked surprised. "A lawyer? Why? I didn't do anything wrong. Besides, I don't know any lawyers here in Ocean City."

"Then I'm sure Mr. Bower here on my left can recommend several." He nodded toward Bower.

"Secondly, you can expect to be contacted by members of the press." He deepened the furrows lining his forehead. "You should be wary of these people. They'll cause problems if they can, both for you and for us. They won't be fair, they'll quote you out of context, and you should treat them as adversaries. My best advice is that you should avoid them completely if you can. We won't discuss the details of these proceedings, and we would suggest that neither should you. When the press calls, it would be best if you declined to talk with them altogether. You should refer them either to Ms. Morse or to your lawyer, when and if you get one. Is that understood?"

"You're ordering me not to talk to the press? You can't do that."

Something flashed behind Bolam's eyes. "Third, as you must have guessed, we've informed the police about this incident. I don't want you to misunderstand; this action wasn't a prejudgment on our part. It wasn't a judgment at all; it was merely a necessary step that needed to be taken for the protection of our institution."

"I don't have anything to hide," Carrie answered. "As I said, I didn't do anything wrong." She tossed her hair, sat poker straight in her chair, and tried to keep up her false veneer of confidence, but it was starting to crack. *Did she do anything wrong?* Now she wasn't so sure.

"Very well, I'd imagine that they'd contact you later this evening.

"Fourth, and this is very difficult for me." He slowed the

cadence of his speech. "I'll need to ask you for your resignation from our house staff."

Carrie visibly recoiled. She hadn't expected that. She'd had a perfect record, and this would ruin it. She wanted to look away, but she knew that she couldn't.

"Under the circumstances we really have no other choice; I hope you understand. It's nothing personal. You should think of it as a temporary measure, one that can be reversed just as soon as the investigation is completed."

Before Carrie could speak, he said, "Fifth, the State Licensing Board will have to be notified. We'll do it first thing on Monday. They'll review your credentials along with our findings. They'll contact the university." Carrie's mouth dropped slightly open. She tried to swallow, but her throat was so dry that nothing much happened. "There's nothing we can do about this," he said. "We're required by law to report potentially wrongful deaths to that body. They may want to talk to you about the status of your license to practice medicine.

"Sixth ..."

"Sixth?" Carrie had had enough. "Hold on a minute. What's going on here?"

"Dr. Williams," he interrupted, "please listen to me. Bill Bennett is going to press charges. There's nothing we can do. We have to protect the hospital."

Carrie just looked at him. The room was silent. All eyes were averted except Bolam's. He stared back at her for a few moments and then again said: "Sixth ..."

But Carrie was no longer listening. She heard his voice but not the words. The signals from her ears somehow got lost on their way to her brain. The sounds were mushy. It was as if he were speaking in a foreign language. *Is this what it's like to have a stroke?* The proceedings continued.

:   :   :

Carrie sat alone in the Sisters of Mercy parking lot, her eyes closed and her head leaning back against her headrest. Rain spattered on the vinyl top of her old 1971 Porsche. It had been her mother's car, but that was a lifetime ago. Now it was hers.

She'd promised herself that she wouldn't cry. It had been the worst day of her life.

What had just happened? Who'd done this thing to her, and why? She'd been deliberately set up and selected as a tool for murder. It made her feel dirty. It was all so far beyond belief that it was unfathomable.

The inquest was over. She'd been banished from the hospital. Dr. Bennett had joined the proceedings. He'd been incredulous, then furious. "Someone pretending to be *me* asked you to kill my patient? That's outrageous."

The chief of staff had suspended her hospital privileges on the spot and had warned her that her medical license was in jeopardy.

She'd become a person of interest in an Ocean City Police Department homicide investigation. Sergeant Willie Tindall had called her and told her so. He'd warned her, "Please keep us apprised of your whereabouts."

"Are you going to arrest me?" Carrie had asked. "Does this mean that I can't leave town?"

"As I said, please keep us apprised of your whereabouts."

Twelve hours ago she'd been a medical superstar, one of the

university's best—they'd told her so. Now people avoided her like a bad case of herpes. It was surreal. It was a nightmare. It was ... .

There came a tap on her car window. An old woman with scraggly gray hair stood just outside her door. She wore at least three layers of dirty, wet clothes, and she motioned for Carrie to roll down her window. "Got a light?" A rain-soaked cigarette bounced up and down in her lips as she talked.

Carrie lowered the window a crack. "Uh, no, sorry." Rain sprinkled in on her shoulder.

The old woman shrugged, and then just as Carrie reached to roll it back up, she said, "Say, I know you." Recognition flashed across her face. "You're the doctor that killed that guy. Your picture was just on TV. I saw it in the lobby."

Carrie didn't know what to say.

The old woman smiled a toothless smile. "That's OK. Old Mary Anne Pinkerton won't tell nobody you're out here." She scratched the right side of her neck with her dirty fingernails. "Men are no damn good. They only want one thing. You did right as far as I'm concerned." She stuck her little finger in her ear and twisted it from side to side. "Kill 'em all. That's what I say."

So now Carrie's photograph was on TV, probably a file photo from the hospital. This could only get worse. "I've got to get out of here," she said to herself. She rolled up her window and started the engine.

Stewart Wolf had been murdered, and she was the only suspect. Her alibi was crazy; even she had trouble believing it. Things were rapidly moving beyond her control. She'd become a victim, and she hated it. She needed to take charge, but how? Where to start?

Wolf and the impostor were her only leads, and Wolf was dead. The woman who claimed to be Wolf's wife was gone, and nobody else had seen her. That was probably a dead end. The assisted-suicide paper trail in Wolf's hospital chart was missing. She shifted into first gear, started out of the parking lot, and found herself literally driving on a road to nowhere. That was unacceptable. She needed a plan, a direction, a hope—anything to clear her name. Moments later, a set of headlights a block and a half away winked on and started to follow.

:  :  :

The rain continued, so Carrie turned on her windshield wipers, whisking away the drops on her windshield. Clouds above her head clung low to the hills. Streetlights sparkled against the gray-black background of a building Pacific storm. The Columbia River was outlined in the distance, and wind blowing in from the west against its current churned its waters like an old-fashioned washing machine.

Carrie babied her car's finicky synchromesh transmission into second gear. The streets were almost deserted and were slick with the rain. She noticed the headlights behind her but didn't think anything of it as they slowly began to close the gap between them. They appeared, disappeared, and then reappeared as she negotiated the curves down toward the river.

She shifted into third. The RPMs dropped below 2,000 as she slowly increased her speed. A dog barked somewhere. Then it barked again. Carrie looked around. She checked her mirrors. It was dark between the streetlights. For some reason, maybe a hangover from the inquest, maybe something else, she felt a sense of unease. She was alone on the road. Rain turned to drizzle but continued to fall.

She drove onto Jackson Street and then over to Jones. Suddenly the headlights were there again. She could tell it was the same car. Was it following her? They trailed, but now at a constant distance. Their reflections came and went in her rearview mirror.

Carrie accelerated, shifted gears, and then accelerated again. She turned a hard left onto Elm Street. The trailing headlights disappeared. Now there was only the empty street behind her, and it glistened in the rain. She smiled to herself and tried to relax. *Silly girl.* Then they reappeared again at the same distance as before.

She slowed her speed to see what would happen. The car behind her slowed. She accelerated to a few miles per hour over the speed limit. The car behind her matched her pace. She turned right, then left, and then right again. The other car traced her turn for turn.

*OK, fine, let's see if you can do this.* She flexed her fingers on the steering wheel. She glanced into her mirrors, double-clutched a downshift back into second, and then stomped the accelerator all the way to the floor. Her car's response was instantaneous. It transmitted its familiar sensation of tightly bridled power and took off like an orange comet.

Carrie shifted into third. She accelerated, braked hard, slid through a left turn, eased up a bit, downshifted, and then turned again. The headlights behind her faded into the distance, and then they winked out. The road behind her was dark, and they were gone.

She cranked her wheel hard onto the Columbia River Highway. Still there was no sign of the following car. She upshifted through the gears. Her speed moved through eighty, ninety, and then one hundred miles per hour. Her engine screamed each time her tachometer approached the red line. And then she saw the headlights again in the distance.

*What's going on here?*

She was on the straightaway now, and her sports car's agility was no longer an advantage. It was power against power, and the car behind her seemed to be gaining.

Suddenly a pair of eyes appeared out of the night, directly in front of her. They reflected the beams from her headlights as two iridescent glistening dots. They blinked on and off as she bore down on them. A deer was on the road. It froze in place. She hit the brakes, but she was going too fast; there was no time to stop. As she swerved hard to the right, her car momentarily lost its traction. It fishtailed around on some loose gravel. Though she fought for control, she went into a four-wheel slide. Tires screeched. Rubber burned. Her car slowed, and then she saw the turn-off to a county road.

She double-clutched a downshift as she turned her wheel, and then double-clutched again. She tapped the brakes, drifted into the turn, then accelerated to counter the centrifugal force. She felt her rear wheels bite into the pavement—she had traction and control again.

She drove a few hundred yards down the spur road and then braked and cut her lights. The car behind was closing fast at a ninety-degree angle. She could hear its engine; it sounded powerful. Its approaching headlights grew large as they cut a path through the night. And then it passed. It roared by in a blur of light and sound. It sped down the road, and she watched it fade into the distance.

When Carrie relaxed her grip on the steering wheel, her fingernail marks were gouged into its leather. She felt shaky. She looked at her hands; they *were* shaky. She'd had an adrenaline surge. She stared at the empty road behind her, thinking, *Is somebody after me?* She reached for her mobile phone and called Candy Peterson, one of her few real friends in Ocean City.

:  :  :

After hearing her story, the first thing Candy said was, "Don't you think that you're getting just a little paranoid? I know you've had a tough day and all, but somebody's after you? Really?" She paused and then answered her own question. "Come on, Carrie. I don't think so! It was probably just a couple of kids out having a good time at your expense. They do it all the time around here. You need to relax a little." Then she asked her if she was OK.

"I'm okay," Carrie answered, "At least I think I'm OK. I'm just tired of people trying to intimidate me, that's all." They talked a while, Carrie's pulse rate returned to normal, and then she changed the subject and asked her about the impostor.

"I remember him," Candy said. "Tall, fit, good-looking. You don't see guys like that around here every day. I'd never seen him before." She paused for a second. "Are you sure you're okay? Do you want me to come over to your place? We could talk, put our heads together about the guy. I'm in a grocery store not five minutes away from your apartment. I could buy a bottle of wine."

"That'd be great, but let's skip the wine. That's the last that thing I need."

They agreed to meet at her apartment in ten minutes. Corroborating the existence of a tall, good-looking man on the seventh floor wasn't much to go on, but at least it was a start.

Carrie stepped on the accelerator. Twelve minutes later she arrived. When she got there, she wasn't at all prepared for what she saw.

Carrie's apartment was half of an old clapboard duplex, the second building in a row of three that hung on a hillside overlooking the Columbia River. Candy waited on the porch as she pulled in. Her expression seemed nervous. As Carrie got out of the car, Candy pointed to the door. It hung ajar. "I haven't been inside yet. I wanted to wait until you got here." Together they peeked in through the doorway and took a collective breath. Candy said, "You can forget about the paranoid comment."

The place was a total wreck. The couch had been tipped upside down, and its cushions were strewn all over the room. The cushions had been cut open, and much of the foam filler had been pulled out. Foam rubber was everywhere. The muslin covering the underside of the couch was ripped down the center, exposing its wooden frame. Two overstuffed chairs were in the same condition, one of them lying beneath a large gouge in the wall. A small side table lay tipped over and broken, its single drawer pulled out and thrown in a corner. The contents of the drawer had been spilled onto the floor and were scattered about. A table lamp and telephone were also on the floor; the lamp was broken, and the telephone cord had been pulled out of the wall. A large mirror had been ripped from its spot and lay smashed below the front window. A cheap French Impressionist print had been torn from its frame. It also lay on the floor, discarded in a corner.

"What do you think happened in here?" Candy asked. "A burglary?"

"I wish that's all that it was," Carrie answered, trying to control the quaver in her voice. She looked around the room. "Somebody was after something, something specific. I think the place has been tossed."

:    :    :

Carrie stepped in over the threshold, but Candy pulled back from the door. "Are you sure we should go in there? Whoever did this could come back."

Instead of responding, Carrie scanned the space in front of her. She bent over and picked up an overturned lamp by its neck. The bottom had been cleanly broken off to reveal its hollow interior.

Another step inside revealed that the kitchen was as bad as the living room. All of the drawers had been pulled out of their cabinets, and their contents had been dumped onto the floor. Broken plates, glasses, and cups were everywhere. Silverware had been tossed into a corner. The oven door was open. A corked quarter-full bottle of wine lay in front of the refrigerator. When Carrie opened the refrigerator door, she saw a milk carton lying on its side and a pool of spilled milk below the bottom shelf. The rest of the refrigerator's contents had been pushed around and out of place.

"Carrie?" Candy remained at the door. "Come on; let's leave. We should get out of here."

"Just a minute," Carrie answered. She turned toward the bedroom. The bedroom door was open, and the bed had been ripped apart. Its mattress and box springs had been pulled off their frame and were askew on the floor. Dresser drawers had been pulled out and discarded, and her clothes had been strewn all over the place. And that's when it hit.

It wasn't the devastation. It was the probing, the determined probing, the searching of her most private possessions. Her hands started to shake. Carrie called back to Candy. "I think you're right. We should leave."

"Damn straight," Candy shouted back. "Now you're talking. Let's hurry up and get out of here."

"Hold on just a second." Carrie picked up her suitcase and surveyed her scattered clothes. She selected a few and then carried the whole bundle out to the porch.

On the way out she glanced in the bathroom. The medicine cabinet had been emptied into the sink, the shower curtain ripped down and the rod removed, the back lid pulled from the toilet, the flotation ball ripped out and opened, and the seat pulled up.

She ran the rest of the way back to Candy.

"You'll need a place to stay," said Candy, closing the door behind her. "You can stay with me if you want, at least for a while."

"Thanks, Candy, but you shouldn't get mixed up in this, at least not more than you already are. There's something going on here that neither one of us understands, and it involves a murder. I may be in danger. I think it best that I disappear for a while."

"Disappear? Really?"

"Really. And I don't want *anyone* to know where I am."

"But the police—"

"I know. I'll tell them later. I *want* the police to be involved with this. I may need their protection. But in the meantime I'd appreciate it if you wouldn't tell anybody about what happened here, at least for now. The press will find out soon enough anyway. Until then, it'll give me time to think, maybe figure all this out a little." They started down the front steps. "And, Candy," she said when they reached the sidewalk, "thanks for being a friend." She kissed her on the cheek.

"But what about—"

Carrie put her index finger on Candy's lips to shush her. "Your friendship means a lot to me." Then she took her suitcase to her car and drove off.

# Chapter 4

JON'S CLOCK RADIO sounded at four. KIRO's DJ wanted to know whether the government was really hiding aliens from the Andromeda galaxy in Roswell, New Mexico. He fumbled for the controls. Karen curled up into a fetal position and pulled her pillow tight around her head. They'd long since made up. She was now nothing but a series of soft mounds and curves under the covers.

Jon crawled out of bed. It was dark outside, and it was cold. The sun wouldn't come up for another three-and-a-half hours. He dressed in jeans, a white shirt, a navy V-necked cashmere sweater that Karen had given him last Christmas, and loafers. Then he quickly checked the Internet to see if there was anything new on the Carrie Williams story. There wasn't. Five minutes later he left the house for Ocean City. The trip in his Explorer would take approximately three-and-a-half hours.

The drive down I-5 was dull. Traffic was light, and as Jon approached his destination, he called the *Seattle Times* to get whatever background he could on Carrie Williams. After a short conversation with a computer—press one, etc.—he was connected with Lizzy Carlstrom, another reporter at the city desk.

"Hi, Liz, you're up early." It was 7:20, and although the sun wasn't up yet, there was plenty of light on the eastern horizon.

"Up early?" she questioned. "I'm up late. Collins had me pull an all-nighter for you. I hope you appreciate it."

"I do, I do. What'd you come up with? What can you tell me about the good Doctor Williams? Any skeletons in her closet that I should know about?"

"Not as many as there are in yours."

"What do you know about my closet?"

"Probably more than I should, but getting back to Carrie Williams, she's really something. She's supposed to be some kind of a medical superstar, a real poster girl for the medical school, according to them one of their very best. And although specific numbers are hard to come by, supposedly her IQ's off the charts. She graduated in the top ten percent of her medical school class without breaking a sweat and was awarded the Resident of the Year award in internal medicine before being assigned to Ocean City. Her pre-med grade-point average was 3.7, only average for students making the med school cut. That was probably disappointing for her. She apparently had issues with some of her undergraduate teachers, but she tested an amazing ninety-eighth percentile in her pre-admission MCAT tests. She's hardly the kind of person that would make up a story about an assisted suicide and expect to get away with it. She's way too smart for that."

"So she's smart," Jon said. "Smart people sometimes do stupid things. What else have you got?" He edged over into the passing lane to pass a slow-moving Ford pickup truck.

"Well, let's see. She was born in Kansas City, single mother, no record of a father, or for that matter of a father figure, in the picture. She and her mother moved to Seattle when she was an infant, and she's a product of the Seattle public school system, Garfield High School.

"Her mother, Thelma, was a nightclub singer by profession, jazz. You might remember her. She had quite a following in the Seattle jazz scene. She was accidentally shot about a year ago while performing at the Sunset Club. A stray bullet fired during a street argument crashed through their front window and struck her square in the chest. They never found the shooter. She lingered for almost a month before she died."

"Oh, yeah, I do remember that, the Sunset Club. Weren't they busted for running prostitution a few years back?"

"That's the place. Anyway, Carrie never really got over it. They offered her counseling at the medical school, but she declined; said she didn't need it and wasn't into that sort of thing. She's apparently a bit of a loner."

Jon slowed as he neared the Ocean City limits. He turned down Front Street toward the public docks. "What about alcohol, drugs, that sort of thing?"

"Nothing there that I could find. She's clean in that department."

"And this is what took you all night?"

"Hey, come on, Jon! You know what it's like."

"OK, only kidding. Anything else?" He turned up the hill toward the hospital. It was now only a block and a half away.

"Sure, she's worked as a model for Nordstrom off and on. Apparently she's a real … ."

Jon interrupted, "Hang on a second." He pulled up to the Sisters of Mercy Medical Center parking lot. It was in total chaos. "There's something going on here."

The parking lot was filled with news vans. Three of them were from Portland, and several had their broadcast antennas extended. News crews were setting up for on-the-scene reports. People were milling around everywhere. "Is there anything new on the wire from Ocean City?" he asked. A uniformed woman wearing a yellow reflection vest waved him away from the parking lot entrance. She said something about not being able to park there. He turned away and pulled to the curb. "Something's happened while I was driving down."

"I don't know," Lizzy answered. "I can check if you want. Don't you listen to the news on the radio?"

"Never."

Jon stopped his car. Several reporters were doing their reports with the hospital as a backdrop. "Listen, there are police and reporters all over the place down here. I've got to go. I'll call you back and get the rest of the Carrie Williams stuff later. I need to find out what's happening."

"Jon?" Liz said into her suddenly silent phone. He'd already hung up. She made a face at the disconnected receiver. "You're welcome."

:  :  :

Jon got out of his car. Two reporters seemed to be jostling for position for their televised reports. Three Ocean City police cruisers were parked near the hospital entrance, and an unmistakable unmarked fourth was parked nearby. It was either a crime scene or somebody had just delivered sextuplets. When Jon recognized a reporter from the *Portland Oregonian,* he approached him and asked, "What's going on?"

"Oh, hi, Jon. I didn't expect to see you down here. There's been another murder, a medical records clerk; they're withholding her name until after they notify the family."

"Another murder?"

"Yeah. An intern found her a few hours ago. She was lying by her desk near the medical records room door. Her neck was broken. No sign of a struggle. Someone just snapped it like the proverbial twig."

Jon looked around and then eyed the hospital entrance. Police guards were everywhere, and they were busy keeping people out.

"And that's not all," he continued. "Get this. You know that doctor, the one who claimed she was tricked into the assisted suicide yesterday?"

Jon returned his focus to the reporter. "Carrie Williams?"

"That's the one. Well, guess what. She's disappeared. She's not at home, she's not in the hospital, she's not anywhere that anybody knows of. We understand that the police would like to talk to her. She's got to be a suspect. Here, look at this." He handed Jon a press release. "They just passed these out. It's from the hospital. This is all we've got. So far nobody's talking. The corporate owners have ordered a circle-the-wagons approach, and the hospital staff has totally closed ranks."

Jon looked at the press release. "Uh-huh, OK, so who's got the story?"

"No one, at least not yet. This is it. You're holding it in your hand."

A sly smile crossed Jon's face. He scanned the one-page paper. "This is crap." He looked back at the hospital entrance and then again at the *Oregonian* reporter. "You're sure nobody has anything yet? Somebody reported the murder. Somebody must have something."

"KETV got an interview with the intern who found her, but other than discovering the body, he didn't know much. Everyone else has clammed up. We're all just cooling our heels until they hold a press conference, and that's not scheduled until late this afternoon. I have no idea what those TV pukes are talking about on camera over there. The guards at the entrances are doing a good job of keeping all of us out."

Jon scanned the press release one more time. "Do you mind if I keep this?" he asked.

"Be my guest."

"Thanks." He put it into his pocket. "I'll be back this afternoon for the press conference. Let me know if anything else develops. I'll see you then."

"Sure, Jon, see you later. Share and share alike, right?"

Jon smiled again, and then he backed away and melted into the crowd.

:     :     :

Jon slowly worked his way toward the hospital entrance. The crowd seemed to be growing. Townspeople had stopped by to see what was going on. He pulled out his cell phone as he walked. He dialed 411 and asked the information operator to connect him with the Sisters of Mercy Medical Center in Ocean City. He then asked the hospital operator to connect him to room 487, saying he was from out of town and that he needed to talk with his brother.

"Do you mean Nicole Early?" said the operator. "She's the only person in room 487. Maybe your brother's in another room.

What's his name?"

Jon hung up the phone. He continued toward the entrance and approached one of the uniformed police officers guarding the doors. "My name's Jon Kirk, and my sister's a patient in there," he said. He nodded toward the entrance. "Her name's Nicole Early. She's in room 487. I came down here from Seattle to see her, and I'm having trouble getting through. Is it all right if I go in?"

The patrolman looked him over. "May I see some ID?" Jon showed him his driver's license. He checked it out. "OK, just a minute." He gave it back to Jon. Then he called someone in the hospital on his radio. "Do you have a Nicole Early in room 487?"

Indeed they did.

"OK, Mr. Kirk, you can pass."

Jon's sly smile returned.

:     :     :

The hospital lobby was large, larger than he'd expected for the size of the building. Three five-hundred-gallon saltwater aquariums to his right divided a seating area from the rest of the lobby. A girl wearing a lightweight pink lab coat, the universal uniform of hospital volunteers everywhere, manned an information desk directly across from the entrance. Her nametag read "Darbie," and she eyed him as he walked over to a hospitality cart and poured a cup of coffee from one of the two thermoses sitting on top. A noticeable commotion came from the other end of the hallway to his left. Several people, including a uniformed policeman, were talking and milling around an open door.

Jon sipped on his coffee. He walked over to a coin-operated

newspaper dispenser, bought a copy of the local paper, and worked his way down the hallway toward the commotion and a sign that identified the medical records room. Looking through the crowd in the hall, he found the medical records room sealed with a single strand of yellow crime-scene tape. The tape was placed chest high so that people could easily duck under it if they needed to go inside. Reaching the back of the group, he moved forward a little so that he could see beyond the tape.

The medical records room itself was neat and orderly. The corpse had been removed. There was no blood anywhere that Jon could see. A chalked outline of a body on the floor near the door was the only obvious sign that a murder had been committed. A man was dusting for fingerprints near a storage file at the back of the room, and a second man was standing just inside the crime-scene tape talking to a woman in a business suit standing on the outside.

Jon got out his cell phone and surreptitiously snapped a few photos. He listened to the conversations around him, thought he heard something about a missing hospital chart and medical record, and then approached one of the uniformed police officers with a few questions. "Any witnesses?" he asked. "Anything missing in there?"

"Who are you?"

"Jon Kirk. I work here." The officer scowled. "Who's the victim? There are all kinds of rumors. I bet I know her. I heard her neck was broken."

Jon was told to move on. He snapped another photo before he walked back to the information desk and asked Darbie if she knew what was happening. She said that she did, but that she wasn't supposed to talk about it. He asked her if she knew Dr. Carrie

Williams. She said she didn't. He asked her if she remembered Stewart Wolf's room number.

"Stewart Wolf? Why are you asking me these things?" She popped some bubble gum between her teeth.

"I'm sorry. I should've introduced myself. I'm Jon Kirk, one of Stew's relatives from Seattle. I drove all the way down here this morning to talk to his nurse. We're looking for a little closure, that's all. The family's very upset. His death was a terrible thing, quite a blow. It's been very hard on all of us. I won't take very much of his nurse's time."

Darbie looked him over. "Uh, I don't know. I suppose there aren't any rules against it, but, well, I guess it's OK. Mr. Wolf was on the seventh floor. I don't know the names of the nurses that took care of him. You should ask the ward clerk when you get up there. She should be able to help you, but don't bother them if they're busy."

Jon said, "I'll be careful not to disturb anyone. Thank you, Darbie."

Darbie watched him leave, and just as soon as he reached the elevators, she picked up her telephone and called hospital administration.

:　:　:

Jon exited the elevator on the seventh floor. The ward was quiet, and the hallways were empty. There was no security. A bored ward clerk looked up from her paperwork and watched him approach the nurses' station. Her nametag read Lucy Boots. "Can I help you?" she asked.

"Yes, please. I'd like to talk with Stewart Wolf's nurse. Is she available?"

"Which one?" she answered. "He had several."

"Any of them. Whoever had the most contact, whoever knows the most about his case. Darbie down in the lobby sent me up here."

"That would be Candy Peterson," she said. "I think she's in 712 giving Mr. Sarkowski a bath. She should be finished almost any time now. Do you want me to page her?"

Jon shook his head. "No, that won't be necessary. I'll just wait outside until she's finished. Which way is room 712?"

Lucy pointed the way. "That way. It's halfway down the hall." Jon thanked her. Lucy then went back to her work.

Jon walked down the hall to room 712 and waited. After several minutes he looked back toward the nurses' station but wasn't able to see the ward clerk at her desk. He assumed that she couldn't see him, either. There were only a few people in the hall. He listened at the hospital room's door. Everything was quiet inside. He knocked on the door, then opened it a crack. "Candy Peterson?" he said softly.

There was no response.

"Candy Peterson," he said again, this time a little louder. He heard some rustling inside, but no one came to the door.

"Candy Peterson?" He pushed the door a little further open. "MR. KIRK!"

"JESUS CHRIST!"

Jon jumped back from the doorway. He turned around with a start. A very large black nurse wearing a green scrub suit covered by an unbuttoned white lab coat seemed to have appeared behind him from out of nowhere. Her hands were on her hips. She had a stethoscope draped around her neck.

"Just what the hell do you think you're doing?" she demanded. She was about five feet nine and weighed at least two hundred pounds, maybe two-thirty. She looked solid. Her nametag read Mavis Porter. She had penetrating eyes.

"Me?" Jon asked. He almost ducked to avoid her stare.

"You see anybody else here?"

"I, uh, I came down here, uh, to visit my sister. Nicole Early. She's in room 487. She's expecting me."

"Your sister!" Mavis chuckled. "You must be kidding." She seemed to grow even larger. "You've got to do a lot better than that."

Jon wore his poker face. "Uh, what do you mean?"

"Well, first of all, you're not even on the right floor."

Jon backed up a step. "OK, I'm on the wrong floor. I'm sorry. I made a mistake; mistakes happen."

"You sure did," she said. "And secondly, Nicole Early's black."

"Black? Are you sure?" Jon looked her in the eye. "I always wondered about that. Mom never told me. She's a stepsister."

"Uh-huh," she said. Her eyes narrowed. "Come with me, Mr. Kirk. Ms. Morse called. She thought you might be up here. She wants to see you in her office."

"Who's Ms. Morse?"

"She's the CEO of this hospital. Now come on. There's nothing for you here." She glared at the ward clerk before turning her attention back to Jon. "Sister!" she said to herself. She shook her head and chuckled again. "That's a good one!"

# Chapter 5

MAVIS ESCORTED JON down to the first floor. She walked slightly behind him and to his right, telling him to turn here, turn there, get in the elevator, that sort of thing. Jon did what he was told. He guessed most people did what they were told when Mavis told them to do it. When they reached the administrative offices, Mavis told him to go in. The administrative office complex had an outer office fronting an inner office. There was a seating area to the left. Alexandra Morse was waiting for him when he arrived.

"So you're Jon Kirk." Alexandra Morse stood next to her secretary's empty desk. It was just outside the door to her inner office. "I've been warned about you. I'm Alex Morse." She smoothed her hair and then extended her hand. "The local newspaper guys said that the *Times* might send you down here. And then when security notified me that you were in the hospital, well, they warned me that you're the type that would do anything for a story."

"Ms. Morse." Jon took her hand.

"Alex," she smiled, "please call me Alex. Everybody does." Her brown shoulder-length hair seemed a little windblown.

"All right, Alex," Jon said. "Call me Jon."

"Good, Jon. Come with me." She opened the door to her inner office and walked inside. Jon followed. He wondered where she was leading him, both figuratively and literally, and he couldn't help but notice the way her legs moved inside her skirt as she walked.

Alex's palatial office was decorated in much the same fashion as the boardroom. With its dark wood paneling and its blood-red deep-pile carpeting, it looked like something that might belong to a bishop or a cardinal, not a hospital administrator. Alex made a gesture toward one of the two high-backed gothic-style chairs that were facing her large oak desk. "Please sit," she said.

Jon eyed the chair before he sat. Diffuse rays of light streamed in through half-shaded windows, illuminating particles of dust as they hung in the air.

"Impressive, aren't they?" she said of the chairs. "The sisters left them behind in the chapel. Once I saw them, I knew I had to have them. These church people really know how to do medieval." She moved around behind her desk, glanced at her watch, and sat down. "Now, then, I understand from my nurses that you've been upstairs wandering around our wards." She shook her head and pursed her lips. "Surely you must know that's against the rules." She waited for a response, and when she got none, she continued. "How did you get past the police at the doors? We try hard to protect our patients and their privacy, not to mention their dignity. Don't you think you're pushing it just a little bit?" She kept up her smile.

Jon answered, "Nobody told me about the rules." He sat in his chair and smiled back at her.

"Really," she said. "Well, that may or may not be true, but either way we can't have unauthorized people roaming around our halls. I'm sure you understand. Now if you'll just tell me what you were after in my hospital."

*Your hospital?* "I was working a story, of course. You knew that. That's my job. You have a very well-trained staff; everyone's been very cooperative. Two murders in two days—that's really something, isn't it? You don't see that every day." Jon watched her smile fade.

Alex was about his age. Her athletic figure reflected hours of work in Ocean City's only fitness club. She was dressed in a tailored gray business suit, no blouse, and high-heeled shoes. There was steel behind the soft veneer of her voice.

"I don't suppose you'd care to tell me what you've uncovered so far?" she asked. Jon didn't answer. "No, I suppose not." Her voice hardened. "Well, in that case, please be a little careful with what you print. There are a lot of unsubstantiated rumors going around, and I wouldn't want you to get it wrong. That wouldn't be good for either of us, if you know what I mean. I'd like to help you if I can." She opened the center drawer of her desk and removed a single sheet of paper. "Why don't I start by giving you a copy of today's press release?" She offered him the paper, pushing it across her desk.

Jon took the paper, folded it, and put it in his pocket without looking at it. "I think I've already seen this," he said. "But I'll read it again later just to make sure I haven't missed anything."

"Most of it's been on TV and the local radio stations already anyway." She leaned back against the gothic carving on her chair. "The stories haven't been very flattering."

"They rarely are."

"And that's a shame," she added. "There are so many good things happening here. They need to be reported, too. You should've seen this place before we took it over. It was on its last legs, a real basket case. The community was about to lose one of its biggest employers. Quality was spotty, and the sisters were losing a ton of their parishioners' money. They knew absolutely nothing about running a business.

"Now we're the most cost-efficient hospital in our system, and that's saying a lot. Our quality's first rate, and we're well in the black. We saved this hospital, and we saved hundreds of jobs in the process. That's a story that needs to be reported, too. That's the one nobody bothers to write."

"I'll keep it in mind," Jon said. He reached into his pocket and took out his note pad. "Two murder in two days." He shook his head. "Would it be all right with you if we start with Carrie Williams?"

"So now we're doing an interview?"

"You said you wanted to help." He clicked the end of his ballpoint pen. He waited.

After a moment she said, "Dr. Williams, of course." Her smile was gone. "That's as good a place to start as any. I'll tell you what I know.

"Dr. Williams is a medical resident down here on a contract from the University of Washington. I don't know her personally, but she's supposed to be smart. She's supposedly a good teacher, and I've heard reports that she's popular with her patients. I think she's done some volunteer work with our surviving-spouse organization. We don't yet understand exactly what went on between Dr. Williams and Mr. Wolf, but we're working on it, and I have no doubts that we'll find out sooner or later. We started a formal inquest as soon as we heard about the incident."

"You mean the murder." Jon wrote something down on his

note pad, and then he asked, "Her work record here has been acceptable?"

"Her work record has been exemplary—that is, with the single exception of yesterday's *incident*."

Jon made eye contact and acknowledged her choice of words with a nod. "Any other problems?"

"None at all."

"And there's no doubt that she's responsible for Mr. Wolf's death?"

"None whatsoever.

"She wrote and signed the morphine order in the chart. The handwriting is hers. We have her bedside actions on tape. She personally set the IV flow pump at a lethal level. She freely admits to everything. Believe me, Jon; Carrie Williams killed Stewart Wolf. That's a fact. There's no absolutely doubt about it. The only relevant question is why."

Jon started to say something else but then caught himself. A puzzled look crossed his face. He paused a moment and then asked, "Did you just say that you have her bedside actions with Stewart Wolf on tape? Is that videotape?"

"Digital tape. It's a part of our new automated record-and-verify patient monitoring system. We use it in our intensive-care unit and sometimes with other patients that require intense monitoring."

"Like Mr. Wolf."

"Exactly."

"And I don't suppose that there's any chance I could have a look at it, is there?"

"The system or the tapes?"

"The tapes."

"Not really. It wouldn't be appropriate. It's a part of his medical record. It's privileged."

"I didn't think so." Jon had more questions about the digital videotape. There were obvious privacy concerns, but he decided to let it go for now. He looked down at his notes. "Do you know if Dr. Williams had known Mr. Wolf prior to his admission?"

"No, I don't. That's one of our avenues of investigation."

"And Dr. Bennett?"

"You mean, had she met him previously?"

"Yes."

"She says, and he confirms, that they hadn't previously met."

Jon furrowed his forehead. "Isn't that a little unusual? I mean, this is a small community, and with only one hospital, there can't be that many physicians in town. Wasn't Dr. Bennett Stewart Wolf's attending physician of record?"

"It's not that unusual," Alex answered. "Bennett doesn't have all that many inpatients, and our residents are authorized to act independently. Besides, Dr. Williams is relatively new. It just so happens that Bennett hadn't admitted any other patients during the time interval between when Dr. Williams arrived and when the incident in question occurred. He's only one of a number of local physicians that rarely interact with our house officers."

"House officers?"

"Interns and residents."

Jon was getting a headache. It had been a long morning, and he needed more caffeine. He rubbed his forehead. "OK," he said slowly. He looked down at the note pad in his left hand. He flipped through a page or two and then asked, "What about friends? You said she was popular with her patients. Did she have many friends on the medical staff? Are there people sticking up for her?"

"I don't know that she has any close friends at all on the medical staff. She seems to be a bit of a loner. She never really fit in very well with the group here. She is, however, close to two of our nurses, Candy Peterson and Mavis Porter. You've met Mavis."

"Oh, yes, I've met Mavis."

"But as for the medical staff ..."

Jon waited for an elaboration. None came. After a pause he asked, "Anything I should know about Dr. Bennett?"

"He's a long-time resident of Ocean City and has a good reputation. There's no problem there."

Jon continued to look at the note pad. Their conversation wasn't leading anywhere, and it wasn't helping his headache. "What do you know about Stewart Wolf?"

"What about him?"

"Well, who was he? Where did he live? How long has he lived in Ocean City? What did he do for a living? What about his wife? What's she like? Did he have any friends? Was his medical condition really incurable? Did he really want to die?"

Alex chuckled and then answered, "Mr. Wolf moved to Ocean City roughly four years ago. He came out here from somewhere back East; I'm not sure exactly from where. To my knowledge he had no family, at least none that we've been able to find. I don't know about his friends. And about his wife—as far as we know, he wasn't married. I have no idea whether he wanted to die or not."

Jon looked back up into Alex's face. "He wasn't married?"

"Not to my knowledge."

"So the story about his wife ..."

"In all probability it isn't true."

"If he wasn't married, why would Dr. Williams … ?"

"I have no idea."

Jon shook his head. The whole thing was crazy. "What about his medical condition?"

"As you know," she said, "he had an incurable brain tumor and only had a short time to live. He wasn't in pain, but there were plenty of other problems. I believe Dr. Williams was sincere when she said she was only trying to help him preserve what little dignity he had left. Assisted suicide has been legal in this state for some time."

"But this wasn't assisted suicide."

"Possibly not."

Jon was running out of questions. He paused a moment before continuing. "Why don't we fast-forward and talk about this morning's *incident* for a few minutes?"

"I'm afraid I can't tell you much about that," she said, "at least not right now. The police have a press conference scheduled for four o'clock this afternoon. We've been asked not to release any information until then."

"OK, I understand, but what about the victim's name?"

"There are family considerations. It'll be released at the press conference."

"And a motive?"

"I wouldn't know. You should ask the police at the press conference."

"Could the two murders, the one yesterday and the one this morning, possibly be connected? After all, Carrie Williams has disappeared, hasn't she?"

"Come on, Jon. The press conference is at four o'clock." Alex painted her smile back on her face.

"I see." Jon smiled back. "Well, then, I guess that's just about it. You've been very helpful. Thank you for your time." He started to stand.

"Write something nice about us," she said. "And be careful about what you may have heard from members of our staff. As I said, there are a lot of unsubstantiated rumors going around. We do good work down here, and we could use a little good press for a change."

"I'll do what I can." He smiled again. He took a step toward the door. Alex stood up as well. "By the way," he said on the way out, "when I was down by the medical records room, I saw that the police were dusting for fingerprints near the storage files. One of them was talking about a missing medical chart. That wouldn't be Stewart Wolf's medical record, would it?" Alex's smile immediately faded into something else. "And you said that the digital videotapes of his hospitalization are a part of his medical record. I assume they were kept in the records room with the rest of his file. Were they taken, too? Could there be something on those tapes that somebody doesn't want us to see?"

Alex stopped short just for a moment but then recovered quickly. She said, "I'm sorry, Mr. Kirk, I really can't respond to that. Maybe at the press conference ..." But she already had responded; her body language told Jon everything he needed to know.

"Well, then, thanks again," he said. "If I have any further questions ... ?"

Alex regained her composure. "Please call," she said. "All the other reporters do."

"I'll keep that in mind," he answered. Then he opened the door and left the room.

# Chapter 6

CANDY PETERSON WAS dispensing medications to Herman Sarkowski, one of her more irascible patients, when she heard the page; she had a telephone call. Someone was holding for her on line four. She walked back to the nurses' station and picked up the phone in the back near where the patient charts were kept. "This is Candy Peterson." She heard a semi-whisper on the other end of the line.

"Candy, it's Carrie. What's going on over there? I just heard about the murder."

Candy turned toward the wall. She cupped her hand around the receiver to shield her voice. "Carrie, where are you? Everyone's looking for you. The police have been up here."

"The police? They don't think I had anything to do with it, do they?"

"I don't think so." She looked over her shoulder to see if anyone was watching. "Where'd you go after we left your apartment last night?"

"I think it's best if you don't know," she answered. "You can't tell anyone if you don't know, and you won't have to lie if they ask. Don't worry; I'm safe, at least for the moment."

"But ..."

"I'll tell you about it later; now tell me about the murder. Was it a robbery? What happened?"

Candy answered, "I'm not sure. They won't tell us anything, but there are rumors. I think it was Linda. They broke her neck."

"They broke her neck? Oh, my God. Why?"

"I don't know. They're keeping us in the dark." Candy again checked to see if anyone was listening. "They found her on the floor by her desk in medical records."

"Medical records?" There was a pause. "What were they after? Was anything missing? I don't really know Linda, but I can't imagine she was a target by herself, not while she was working in the hospital. God, I hope they weren't after Stewart Wolf's chart. That would tie this to me."

"Carrie, I don't know anything. They warned us not to talk to anybody. Everyone's on edge. There's going to be a press conference this afternoon. Maybe they'll tell us something then.

"Listen, Carrie, I think you should call the police. Tell them where you are. Talk to them; tell them you didn't have anything to do with this. Tell them about your apartment. They can protect you. When someone messed up your apartment last night, they were searching for something. And now there's Linda. I'm really scared for you. Call the police. We all know you're innocent."

"No, no police." Carrie was emphatic. "I can't do that, not now. Don't you see what's going on here? The killers are tying up loose ends. They used me to kill Mr. Wolf. They probably killed Linda to get to his medical chart. And now I have to be next on their list. I'm a loose end, a loose end that needs to be tied up. The police will want me to come back to Ocean City, and I can't do that. It's too dangerous for me there. There's no way they can protect me from people like this. I'm safe here where I am, at least for now. I need to hide."

Candy paused and then said, "You're in danger, and you don't want to call the police? Carrie …"

"Look, Candy, I know how strange this whole thing must seem, but I'm a little stressed right now. I just need some time."

"But no police?"

"No police."

Candy checked over her shoulder. Now the ward clerk looked as if she might be listening to her conversation. She turned back toward the phone on the wall and lowered her voice to a half-whisper. "Carrie, what's going on here? Really? Is there something you're not telling me? You can tell me. I won't tell anybody."

Carrie didn't answer right away, then said, "I know I owe you more of an explanation, and I don't blame you for having questions. It's just that there's nothing more I can say right now. OK?" There was silence on the other end of the line. "OK?"

"OK, Carrie, have it your way, but just one thing. When you're free to talk, when you're done with all of this, whatever it is, you'll tell me what it's all about, won't you? I think you owe me at least that much."

"I owe you more than I could ever possibly repay," Carrie replied. "You're a great friend." And then she added, "But as I already told you, I have no idea what this is all about."

Then Carrie asked her for a big favor.

# Chapter 7

JON STOOD IN LINE in the cafeteria waiting to get the caffeine he needed to help his headache. What had he just learned?

The Stewart Wolf and medical-records-clerk murders were undoubtedly connected, and Carrie Williams had to somehow be connected to both. Carrie was a loner and had only two close friends in the hospital, Candy Peterson and Mavis Porter, both of whom were nurses. Both worked on the seventh floor, and both took care of Stewart Wolf. Wolf's medical records, including the digital tapes of his hospitalization, were in all probability stolen, and the theft was likely the motive for the clerk's death. And what was on the tapes? They would have shown Carrie administering the drugs that killed Wolf, but what else? It would have taken a strong person to snap the records clerk's neck, someone who knew how to do that kind of work. Carrie couldn't have done that, could she? Had she had some sort of martial arts training, or something else?

The electronic media had already reported what was known about the murders. Jon needed a different angle. He needed to verify facts and get something fresh. He needed to get back to the seventh floor and talk with Candy Peterson. He moved on past the plastic bowls filled with yellow-and-green Jell-O to the large stainless-steel coffee container at the end of the line. The coffee looked thin and watery as he splashed it into his extra-large Styrofoam cup. He looked down and imagined he could see all the way through it to the bottom. "Is this Starbucks?" he asked the cashier.

"What? Regular coffee's not good enough for you?" said a familiar voice immediately to his back. He winced when he heard it. He turned around to see Mavis Porter standing behind him. She'd brought her own personalized coffee cup with her. It was white with a red thermometer enameled on the side. A caption under it stated in bold black letters, "UP YOURS."

"You did it again. Don't do that," Jon said.

"Don't do what?"

"Don't sneak up on people like that."

"The way I remember it, you're the one that's been doing the sneaking," she said. "You find what you came for?"

Jon paid for his coffee. "What are you talking about, Mavis?"

"You're a reporter. You came down here to find out about Carrie and the murders, didn't you? Poor little black girl in trouble with the law. Well? Did you get what you came for?" She topped off her cup with black coffee.

"I don't know."

"Didn't think so," she grunted. "Some reporter." She moved up to the cashier.

"Mavis," he asked, "what have you got against me, anyway?"

She turned to look at him. "Well, for one thing," she said, "you're standing in my way." Jon stepped to the side, and she paid the cashier. "For another, you went wandering around on my ward without my permission. I don't like that. And for a third, you're going to write a nasty article about a nice woman doctor from Seattle that you know nothing about."

"You don't know what I'm going to write." They moved away from the cashier.

"Oh? I suppose you're different from all those other reporters," she said. "You must not have seen the morning paper. Young African-American woman doctor disappears after killing patient."

"I saw it," he said, "at least the headline. The electronic media had it, too."

"Then you know we're all a bunch of dumb hicks out here. We run a loose ship. We don't know anything about high-tech medicine or quality control. We'd really be in deep doo-doo if the Hospital Corporation of North America hadn't bought us out and saved our collective asses. Give me a break!" Her stare penetrated his practiced defenses, and when she broke through, she did it in a dismissive sort of way.

"Look, Mavis," Jon said. "If you've got something to say, I'll listen. If you have information about Carrie Williams and it's relevant, I'll use it. Otherwise, we should probably end this conversation. My coffee's getting cold."

"Um-hum," she said, looking him up and down.

"Um-hum what?"

She made a harrumph sort of noise.

"Come on, Mavis … ."

"Listen," she said. "Those other reporters got it wrong. There's no way that Carrie Williams did what they say she did. No way! That girl doesn't lie." She switched her coffee into her left hand and pointed her right index finger at Jon's chest. "Somebody's trying to take that girl down. She doesn't deserve this." She pointed again for emphasis, this time touching his shirt. "And if I ever find out who it is … ." She took a deep breath. "'There's lots of funny stuff going on around this place."

Jon looked down at her finger, then back up at her face. His jaw was clenched. She retracted her hand. "What do you mean, Mavis?" When she didn't answer right away, he asked, "What sort of funny stuff?"

"How was your interview with Alex Morse?" She answered his question with a question. "Did she tell you how efficient we are now and how they saved us all from bankruptcy and made us the most profitable hospital in the system? Did she tell you about all the jobs they saved? Did she tell you all of that? I'll bet she did."

"She told me that you and Candy Peterson are Carrie's best friends."

"Well, at least she got one thing right."

"And she told me about an inquest."

"The inquest? Hah! That's a laugh. All they're interested in is damage control."

"You don't think they're after the truth?"

Mavis tilted her head to the side. "Are you interested in the truth, Mr. Kirk? Do you really want to know what's going on around here? Are you an honest reporter? Is there such a thing?"

"Come on, Mavis, don't be so hostile. Tell me about the 'funny stuff'. I think we're both on the same side here. There've been two murders in this place in two days. Carrie Williams claims she's been used as the murder weapon in the first. It's an incredible claim, and nobody believes her."

"I do."

"Yes, I know. You said that. But now there's been a second, and she could be blamed for that one, too. The two are undoubtedly tied together. It's all a part of the same plot against her. Your friend's in serious need of some help."

She raised an eyebrow. "What do you mean by that?"

"OK, well, I have reason to believe that the clerk in medical records was killed so that someone could steal Stewart Wolf's medical chart, including the digital tapes that were made of his hospital stay. There must've been something on those tapes that either the killer desperately wanted to see or desperately didn't want other people to see. The murders are obviously connected. People are going to start connecting the dots, and those dots are going to point directly at Carrie.

"Come on, Mavis; let me help your friend. If she's as innocent as you say she is, I'll do everything in my power to clear her name. I give you my word.

"Tell me about the funny stuff."

Mavis paused a moment and then said, "You know about the tapes? Ms. Morse told you about that?"

"I don't think she meant to. She mentioned it in passing. She stonewalled me for most of the interview."

"Yeah, she's good at that. Candy knows more about those tapes than I do. I don't really understand the purpose of the system, anyway. It hasn't been used with any other patient."

"So Wolf was the first?"

"The one and only as far as I know." She paused another moment and then asked, "You really think that Linda, that's the records clerk, was murdered for the tapes?"

"That's how it looks to me at this point. Let's work together on this. We both want the same thing. We both want the truth to come out. Tell me what's going on around here."

"You're going to write about it the way I tell it?"

"I will if it's accurate and if it can be verified."

"All right, Mr. Kirk, you've got a deal, and don't think I won't hold you to it. Now about Carrie ..."

"She gets a fair break. If she's telling the truth, I'll work hard and use the power of the press to clear her name. If not, well ..."

Mavis slowly nodded her head. "Come with me. I've got something to show you. Dump your coffee." She poured hers in a trash receptacle. "Before you write anything, there are things you ought to know about this place." She started down the hallway. Jon threw his coffee away and followed.

"What things?" he asked.

"Things," she said. "Things you didn't ask Alex Morse but should have. Things the other reporters either ignored or don't know. Important things."

He hurried to keep up. "How would you know what I asked Alex Morse?"

Mavis abruptly stopped and turned sideways to face him. Jon stopped as well. She locked on to his eyes with her own. "You asked her about Stewart Wolf, didn't you?"

"Of course."

"So she told you he was a consultant to this hospital, a financial consultant."

"Uh, I'm not sure that she mentioned that."

"Bet you didn't ask her about the body."

"The body?" he questioned.

"Yeah, the body. You know, Stewart Wolf's body."

"Huh?"

"Did you ask her what happened to it?" Jon just looked at her. "He doesn't have any relatives, you know. No wife, no one to take care of things." Jon wasn't sure what to say. "Didn't think so," she said. "Come with me." She led Jon through the lobby and onto an elevator.

"Where're we going?"

"You'll see." She pushed the button labeled *B*. "We'll be there in a minute or two."

"If we're going to the morgue, I'll pass," Jon said. He had a thing about dead bodies and morgues. He'd once passed out during an autopsy in front of Karen, and she'd never let him forget it. He didn't want to repeat the experience with Mavis.

"We're not going to the morgue," she said.

When they reached the basement, they got off the elevator and walked to an unmarked door about sixty feet down the hall. Mavis unlocked the door with her charge-nurse master key. They stepped inside. In a small all-glass sterile room within a room, technicians wearing surgical masks and dressed in surgical garb were standing around a stainless-steel table. Mavis nodded to the technicians. One of them nodded back. The others were concentrating on their work. They were standing around the table, meticulously, slowly, and methodically stripping the skin away from a male body. The top of his head had been removed, exposing an empty cranial cavity. His brain was gone. A long L-shaped cut had been stitched together with heavy black sutures extending from his chest to his pelvis. His legs had been skinned to his ankles, and his arms had been skinned to his wrists, creating the impression of bare muscles wearing mottled leather gloves and boots. The technicians were working on his abdomen. A sign over an all-glass inner door read:

*Sterile Environment*
*Positive Pressure Air Flow*

"Let me introduce you to Stewart Wolf," she said. "The next thing they're going to do is to pull out his bones."

Jon felt the blood drain from his face. His heart started to pound in his chest. "What the hell is that?" He blinked his eyes and was suddenly lightheaded.

"Money," she said. "Lots of money."

A few of the technicians looked up for a moment and then went back to their work.

# Chapter 8

"YOU ALWAYS BEEN this squeamish?" she asked Jon. They were back out in the hallway. She leaned against the wall and folded her arms across her ample chest. Jon looked a little pale.

"Blood and guts have never been my strong suit," he answered. He wiped a few beads of sweat away from his forehead.

She shook her head and snorted, "Pathetic." She unfolded her arms and stood away from the wall. "Come on. Let's get out of here. We'll go back to the cafeteria and get you your coffee. You look like you could use it."

They walked to the elevator, rode it back up to the main floor, and then walked back to the lunchroom. Jon bought their coffee while she refilled her *UP YOURS* cup. Then they went over to a quiet table in a corner and sat down. She said, "Let's talk." A man in a hospital gown pushing an IV pole shuffled away.

"OK, Mavis," Jon said, "you got my attention. Now what was that all about?" The color was starting to return to his face.

"That, Mr. Kirk, is how this place has become the profit-making star of the corporate hospital world. And despite what Ms. Alex Morse may have told you, efficiency of operation has nothing to do with it. This is just one of their little secrets. It was

Stewart Wolf's idea." She looked down at her coffee mug, blew across the top, and then took a sip.

"Whoa." He reached into his pocket, pulled out his note pad, and put it on the table. "You're telling me they sell organs for profit? Come on. That sounds like something from an old Robin Cook novel."

"Yeah, I saw the movie," she said. "It wasn't that bad. But, no, they don't sell organs. That's illegal. They would if they could, mind you, but they can't. They bend the rules here as far as they can, but they don't break them. They're careful about that. That's the way Wolf set it up. But these new owners would do anything to make a buck." The man with the IV pole bumped into a table with a clank.

"They're processing parts," she continued. "Not just the organs you usually think about for transplants, but all body parts. There's a big difference. It's a chop-shop type of operation."

"Like an auto chop shop?"

"Yeah. My brother, Brian, was into that. He's in jail now. This is almost the same thing, but it's legal. They don't steal the bodies; they get people to donate them."

"And then they sell the parts."

"Almost," she said, "but not quite. It's just as illegal to sell non-organ body parts as it is to sell internal organs, but the regulations are different; they're much more lax. You can charge an unregulated fee to process non-organ body parts, supposedly to cover costs such as dissecting them out of a cadaver, cleaning them, storing them, that sort of thing. Think of it as a shipping and handling charge."

"And that was what they were doing down there in the basement?"

"Bingo!" Mavis touched her nose with her index finger. "You got it. They were processing."

Jon started to write.

"You see," she said, "when the Sisters of Mercy set up the place, they did it to heal the sick and take care of the poor. That was their mission, their goal—their only goal. That was their reason for being. Money was never an issue. They charged people only as much as they could afford, cross-subsidized care for the indigent, and the church took care of the rest. It all worked fine until the cost of medical care exploded. Then the whole thing started to break down." She sipped some of her coffee.

"Medicare reimbursement was cut, and Medicaid rates fell through the floor. Other regional hospitals looked for excuses to offload their no-pay patients in our direction. We, of course, took them all without question.

"Then the church finally threatened to cut off our subsidy, and the whole thing imploded. We almost went bust. And we would have, too, if it weren't for the Hospital Corporation of North America. They rode in on their white horses and saved our collective ass."

The cafeteria cash register whirred in the background as it tallied up the morning's receipts. It was one of those older semimechanical ones that made a lot of noise while it did its work.

"At first we were ecstatic," Mavis continued. "We loved the new owners. They saved our jobs. Then things started to change." She took another sip of her coffee and then put her cup back down on the table. "They brought in an efficiency expert, then a new administrator and a new medical chief of staff. They increased charges where they could and cut nursing levels to the absolute minimum. They automated our labs and radiology. Their x-rays are now read in India. They pushed patients out of the hospital way before they were ready. They all but eliminated our social work department. And then, of course, they got rid of the unions. When Wolf showed up one day and started making suggestions—the for-profit tissue bank was one of them—they really started to roll.

"You getting all this?" she asked.

"Hang on a second," Jon said. He put down his pen and drank some of his coffee. Then he flexed his fingers and picked up his pen again. "OK, go ahead."

"OK," she said. She took a sip of her coffee. "Here's how it works. People die. Most of the bodies come from the hospital, but some come from mortuaries. There's probably some kind of a kickback going on, although I'm sure they'd call it a finder's fee or something. Anyway, the hospital people are responsible for the tissue and organ donations. They get the patients or their families to sign the papers. It's an easy sell, and they're good at it. It's especially easy with assisted-suicide patients."

"Just a minute," Jon said. He wrote something and then asked, "If the tissues are donated, how can they …"

"Charge for them?" She finished his sentence. "They don't. They charge for the processing, remember? And the real crime is that the families don't get a dime of the money. Those guys in the basement peel off skin, cut out heart valves, strip away tendons, scoop out fascia. …"

"Hold it," he interrupted. He scribbled on his note pad until he caught up. Then he looked up and asked, "What's fascia?"

"Subcutaneous connective tissue, the stuff between skin and muscle. They use it to get rid of wrinkles and scars, make pouty lips, stuff like that. With their processing charges, it's worth about two thousand dollars a pop. Anyway, they pull out the bones, harvest the corneas; sometimes they take out the knee joints as a whole. They use as much of the bodies as they can. It's big business, and I'm sure the corporate shareholders love it. They get about a quarter of a million dollars a corpse. Not bad for processing, is it?"

Jon held up his hand. "Just a minute," he said as he kept writing. "They use the skin for burns?"

"And penis enlargements," she said.

"Penis enlargements?" He looked up from his note pad.

"Yeah," she chuckled, "at least for the white guys."

Jon looked at her for a moment or two and then said, "Right." He wrote a little more. "And the bones?"

"They can use them whole as replacements or grind them up to inject as a way to promote healing. They can even machine them into special shapes. Ground-up bone goes for about fifty bucks a teaspoon. They get about twenty-five hundred for tendons and over seven thousand for heart valves. Body-part recycling is a billion-dollar-a-year industry."

Jon wrote that down, paused, and shook his head. Then he looked back up at Mavis. "How do you know all this?"

"I talk to people," she said. "People tell me things. There isn't much that goes on around here that I don't know about."

Jon took a sip of his coffee. He flipped through a few pages of his note pad. "Let's see if I've got this right. Stewart Wolf was a consultant to the hospital, a sort of financial advisor. I'll get back to that in a minute. He'd contracted an incurable form of cancer, was admitted to the hospital, and then a day later was killed, euthanized. According to you, somebody duped Carrie into killing him. Then his body somehow ends up in a tissue recycling lab that he helped create."

"He probably signed his own donation papers when he set up the facility," she said. "I just wanted you to know what goes on around here before you start writing stories critical of Carrie. There's no way she murdered that guy the way they say she did. If she says there was another Dr. Bennett, then there was another Dr. Bennett. That's just the way it is. Your buddies in the press are putting a big hurt on a girl that doesn't deserve it."

Jon scratched his head. "I hope you're right," he said. "Let's see. I was going to ask you something. Oh, yeah, what about the brain? Wolf's skull was empty; at least I think it was. What'd they do with his brain?"

"Nothing," she said. "They scrape the surface to get the membrane that covers it, but the brains themselves are worthless. They probably stuffed it in his abdomen before they sewed it back up. If they left it in his head, it might liquefy, and fluids might leak out. Can't have that at a fancy funeral."

Jon's face again went a little pale.

"You *are* going to write about this, aren't you?" she asked.

"Uh, yeah, I think so. I'd still like to learn a little more."

"The local reporters won't touch it, but somebody should do it. People need to know what goes on around here. You're from out of state. You'd have no reason to keep it quiet. What they're doing may be legal, but it isn't right."

"It's a hell of a way to make money. I've got to agree with you there." Jon put down his note pad, flexed his fingers, and then picked it up again. "Tell me, what's wrong with the local press? What am I missing here?"

"Look around, Kirk. In case you haven't noticed, this town

isn't doing so good. The only thing we've got going here is the Coast Guard station and the hospital, and maybe a little tourism in the summer. Unemployment is high. The hospital employs a lot of people. Nobody wants to rain on our parade; there's enough rain around here as it is."

'No argument there," Jon said. He glanced out the window. Water was running down the outside of the panes in rivulets. "Let's talk about Stewart Wolf." He turned to a new page. "Let's assume for a moment that somebody did set Dr. Williams up. If that indeed is true, then it's Wolf who's central to this whole thing, not Carrie. Exactly who was he, and what was his job with the hospital?"

"I'm not sure," she answered. "I never saw his name on an organizational chart. I don't think he had a real job. He'd just show up from time to time. He seemed to be an accountant or something like that. He knew a lot about money. He was some kind of consultant. He'd offer suggestions, ways to increase profitability."

"Suggestions like the tissue-processing lab."

"Like that, and others. He knew a lot about billing the government for Medicare and Medicaid; he was real smart about that. He knew a lot about their computers. He also got the Pacific Northwest Forensics Laboratory approved and funded by the Justice Department. That's a huge moneymaker."

"The Pacific Northwest Forensics Laboratory?"

"Yeah, it's an FBI operation. Their crime lab runs the place. The hospital leases them the land and supplies them with bodies for their decomposition studies."

"What?"

"Decomposition studies."

Jon winced a bit.

"Yeah! Creepy, isn't it?"

He rubbed his chin. "Mavis, how could you possibly know all of this stuff?"

"Oh, I get around. And by the way, as far as your newspaper's concerned, you heard it from a well-placed unnamed source within the hospital." Her beeper went off. She pushed a button to retrieve the message and then watched it scroll across her LCD. "I've got to go," she said. "We've got a code brown up on the floor." She looked up from her beeper and back at Jon. "You want to come up with me? You wanted to talk with Candy Peterson, didn't you? She knows all about the video system. You can see her while I take care of my patient."

Jon put his coffee down on the table. "Sure. Thanks, Mavis."

"OK, then, let's go."

When they stepped off the elevator onto the medical ward, they were immediately enveloped by a seriously malodorous smell.

"Jesus," Jon asked, "what's that?"

"That's the code brown," she answered. "Herman Sarkowski in 712 shit the bed again. He does that every now and then just to get a little attention. If you ask me, Mr. Sarkowski ought to be the next candidate for assisted suicide around here. I've got to go in and check him out. Why don't you go over to the nurses' station and find Candy? She'll tell you what you want to know."

Jon went to the nurses' station and once more asked the ward clerk if he could speak with Candy Peterson. He was told that Candy had left for the day. She'd received a phone call and abruptly left the hospital before the end of her shift.

# Chapter 9

THE BIG MAN HEARD a key slide into the lock. He was instantly alert. His right hand moved toward the pistol he kept near him at all times. His muscles tensed. His athletic body was ready to do whatever needed to be done. He wasn't heavily muscled like a body builder but instead was built more like a sprinter or a swimmer. His conservatively styled clothes hid three scars, two from large-caliber bullets and one from a serrated fish knife. They bore witness to unsuccessful attempts to take him by surprise in the past. None of his attackers had survived.

The key turned in the lock, the door opened, and his tightly wound muscles uncoiled as his partner walked into the room. She tossed her keys into a dish on a table beside the door. "Did you get it?" he asked her after she shut the door and locked it behind her. The tension in his body continued to dissipate.

"I got it," she answered. "The tapes were where they were supposed to be, along with the rest of his medical records. It went like clockwork, just as we planned it. Piece of cake."

"It took you long enough." He dropped his right hand back to his side, away from his gun.

"I stopped by a Denny's on the way back to get something to

eat. I was hungry. I should've brought you something." She took off her raincoat and shook it out.

"Your collateral damage with the records clerk made the news," he said to her as she tossed her raincoat over the back of a chair. "It's on all the channels. Was that really necessary?"

"It was a contingency that we'd planned for, and it couldn't be helped. Besides, she pissed me off." She brushed the water droplets out of her hair with her fingers.

"Uh-huh, what'd she do, question your parental heritage?"

She answered his question with an extension of her middle finger. Then she took the package she'd been carrying over to a portable card table in the center of the room and placed it down in front of a twenty-four-inch flat-screen TV monitor. The monitor was connected to a set of small audio speakers and hardwired to a digital tape player. She turned the monitor on.

The man closed the lid to his laptop computer and put it aside on a coffee table. Then he stood to join her by the AV equipment. "You know, sometimes I think you enjoy your work a little too much."

"Don't worry; everything's clean, no traces. Anyway, I was half-looking for some kind of a mess to leave behind. It'll keep people distracted, at least for a while. There's nothing like a good murder to keep the local gendarmes busy, busy, busy." She flipped the switch on the digital tape player. The TV monitor flashed on. A solid blue background highlighted white lettering in the upper right corner, indicating no signal from video input #1.

The woman opened her package and dumped Stewart Wolf's hospital chart, registration and insurance documents, and several digital tapes out onto the card table. She sorted through the material in front of her. "We won't be needing this," she said of the hospital chart. "There's nothing in it. I went through it in the car." She pushed it aside. "We should shred it along with the rest of his paperwork after we're finished here." Then she found a tape cassette with the number "1" marked on it. She inserted it into its slot. The lettering vanished from the upper right corner of the video monitor. Then in white letters they saw these words:

SISTERS OF MERCY MEDICAL CENTER
PATIENT: STEWART WOLF
TAPE 1

The man pulled two chairs over in front of the screen. "You ready to do this?"

"Just about." She turned away and started out of the room. "Why don't you sit down? I'll be back in a minute."

"Where are you going?"

"I'm going to the bathroom. Is that OK with you? I've got to take a piss."

The man didn't answer. Instead he sat down, pushed "play," and started to watch tape number 1.

# Chapter 10

CARRIE PEEKED OUT from behind the curtain of her motel room window. She was in serious trouble, and she knew it. First Stewart Wolf and then Linda in medical records—the pattern was clear. She was next on the list. There was no doubt that they were tying up loose ends. She'd tried hard to be careful, but still there was always the possibility that they'd been able to follow her. She'd spent the night in one of those old 1950s-vintage motels that you drive by on the highway but never really see.

After finding her apartment trashed, she'd left town as fast as she could. She'd driven to Portland and then on to the Portland airport. She knew that she'd have to get rid of her Porsche; it was far too noticeable. So she'd pulled her suitcase out of the trunk, locked her car, and then just walked away. She'd hoped that leaving her car at the airport parking lot would cause problems for her pursuers. Once they found it, they'd have to search the airline manifests to see if she'd booked a flight. That would take time, and she was well aware that time was not on her side.

Carrie had walked to a cabstand near the arriving flights area and hired a cab. She'd asked to be taken downtown to Portland's central bus station. From there she'd taken another cab, this time from a different cab company, up the hill to the administrative offices of the Oregon Health Sciences University. The university was a busy place and the home of the state's only medical school, and she knew from past experience that she'd be able to blend in there with the local medical crowd. She'd stood outside the admin building entrance until the cab drove away, then had pulled her suitcase down the hill to the university's shuttle bus stop. There she waited with a group of hospital interns and residents for about twenty minutes until the next shuttle bus arrived. She was headed for Kaiser Permanente Medical Center, the region's largest HMO. When the bus came, she'd boarded and moved to a vacant seat. Then she'd spent the rest of the trip looking down at her shoes, trying to avoid any memorable human contact. The entire trip took approximately twenty-five minutes.

After arriving at Kaiser, she'd walked into the lobby, found a list of free hotel and motel pickup services, selected one, and called for a pickup. She'd checked in under the name of Belle Maxwell and paid cash for one night's stay in a first-floor room with a kitchenette. Once safely inside, with the door carefully locked behind her, she'd crashed on her bed for some much-needed rest. Unfortunately, sleep wouldn't come. After a while she'd made the first of many trips to the window to see if anyone was outside. She'd spent a long, restless night waiting in anticipation for a knock on her door that thankfully never came.

Carrie was nervous. Linda's death had shaken her. She peeked out through the curtains again to see if there was anyone hanging around outside; there wasn't. She checked her watch; it was ten minutes to checkout time. It was time to move on.

She recalled her conversations with Stewart Wolf, the things he'd said after she'd administered the stimulant. Could it all be true? More likely he'd been out of his head.

She called Mavis to find out if she knew anything different from what Candy had told her. Mavis described the media frenzy in their parking lot and her conversations with Jon. She mentioned his theory about the digital tapes. "I think he's one of the good guys," she said. "He says he wants to help. I believe him." Carrie responded that she didn't trust reporters. "You ought to think about his offer," Mavis reiterated. "You could use all the help you can get." Carrie thanked her for the suggestion, asked her to remind Candy to be careful, and then hung up the phone.

Carrie peered out the window once more. The coast was clear. She gathered up her belongings and packed her suitcase for the next leg of her trip. She checked the motel room to make sure that she hadn't left anything behind, then again took out her cell phone and tapped in a number. This time it was a number she'd known by heart since she was a child. The phone rang only once.

"Jussa minute," a gravelly voice said on the other end of the line. The soft sounds of Sarah Vaughn singing "Sophisticated Lady" were playing somewhere in the background. She heard the clacking of the receiver as it was placed down on a table. The music died down, and then the phone was picked up again. "Who's this?" It was the same gravelly voice.

"Chester?" Carrie questioned.

"Carrie? Carrie, is that you?"

"It's me, Chester."

"Carrie, it is you. Goddamn, it sure is great to hear your voice again. You don't know how I've missed that sweet sound. You still singing? I used to listen to you on Sundays, picked your voice up right out of the choir. You had your mamma's voice."

"Thanks, Chester. You don't know how great it is to hear you, too."

"Not so sweet, though, eh? Where you been, anyway? Goddamn, your mamma'd turn over in her grave if she knew how long it's been since you've called."

"My momma'd turn over in her grave if she heard you take the Lord's name in vain like that. You know she would."

"No doubt about that, Carrie, no doubt about that." He chuckled a gravelly chuckle.

Carrie felt comfort in his voice. She'd known him all of her life. He was older, and he'd been her mother's special friend. He'd been a part of her life for as long as she could remember. "Chester," she finally said, "I'm in trouble. I'm in big trouble." She took a deep breath. "I'm in trouble and I really need your help."

He heard the catch in her voice. "What is it, baby?"

# Chapter 11

Sergeant Tindall called the press conference to order and read an opening statement. "At approximately five-fifteen this morning, Linda Ducommun was found dead near her desk in the medical records room … ." The electronic media types in the front rows diligently took notes and preened for the cameras while waiting for their turns to ask brilliant, probing questions. Their TV crews spent as much time taping them as the speaker on the podium.

Jon sat at the back of the room. He was playing a video game on his BlackBerry. He hated the electronic media, its personality cults, and the way their reporters compressed entire news stories into sound bites of only a few seconds each. It was always more about them than about the news. Besides, he'd already finished his story about tissue harvesting and the hospital's finances, and it was a blockbuster. Most of it would be his exclusive. Even the lawyers left it alone. It seemed they particularly liked stories that disparaged the medical professions. He'd filed it in plenty of time to make the next day's paper, and if anything of interest came up at the press conference, he could add it later. Collins liked it, too, but he told Jon he was still waiting for something on Carrie. Jon promised him that that would come later.

"How much later?" he'd asked.

"Soon."

Jon had spent his afternoon checking details. He'd tried to reach Candy Peterson, leaving messages both at her home and on her cell phone. He'd asked her to call or e-mail him as soon as possible. So far there'd been no response. He'd wanted to hear whatever she could tell him about Carrie Williams, and most of all he'd wanted to find out about the hospital's digital-tape patient-monitoring system. He'd made a mental note to call her again just as soon as the press conference was over.

He'd confirmed Mavis's part of the story by calling Alex Morse. Alex had been polite and businesslike, answering all his questions about the human-tissue-processing center. Yes, they made a substantial profit on their tissue-processing operation. No, they didn't inform donors about the money, but under Oregon law they weren't allowed to pay patients or their families for donations of human organs or tissue, anyway. And there was no connection between physician-assisted suicide and the human-tissue-processing center whatsoever. Oregon's death-with-dignity law provided elaborate safety mechanisms, including waiting periods, second opinions, witnesses not related to dying persons—that sort of thing—that ensured against sinister temptations leading down a slippery slope toward euthanasia. The entire program was conducted for the good of all concerned, and there were hundreds of patients, maybe thousands, who now enjoyed an improved quality of life because of the efforts at the tissue bank. They were all proud of the things they'd accomplished at the Sisters of Mercy Medical Center, and certainly he could quote her.

Tindall's opening statement revealed nothing that Jon hadn't already discovered. The family of the victim had been notified, and the investigation was under way. They were awaiting forensic reports from the CSI team on loan from Portland. The motive seemed to be theft; Stewart Wolf's medical records were missing. Nothing else was taken. They had some leads but were unwilling to discuss them at this time. Then he opened it up for questions.

The TV reporters sprang into action. Why were Stewart Wolf's medical records stolen? What was in them that connected this crime to Wolf's death? How could someone get all the way to the medical records room in the middle of the night without being seen? Where was Carrie Williams? Was she a suspect? Could she have been strong enough to break a person's neck? Why hadn't they taken her into custody after the first murder?

Jon checked his e-mail while he half-listened to the proceedings.

*A priest, a rabbi, and a mullah were riding in an airplane ...*
DELETE!

*Bill Clinton and George Bush were sitting in a strip joint when Carol Wright slithered onto the stage with her python.*
DELETE!

*Married women are fatter than single women. Single women come home, look in the refrigerator, and go straight to bed. Married women come home, look in the bed, and go straight to the refrigerator.*

Not bad. Maybe a keeper.

A reporter asked Tindall about potential DNA evidence. Did they have a sample from Carrie Williams? Would that be a way to tie her to the crime scene? As Tindall started to answer, Jon saw a message from candypete@aol.com pop into his mailbox. "*Candypete?*" He sat up in his chair and clicked on the icon.

*Dear Mr. Kirk,*

*You left me a message to call. I don't have my cell phone, and it's not safe for me to go back and get it. It's important that we talk as soon as possible. Mavis said I could trust you.*

*I'm leaving for Seattle immediately; hopefully you can meet me there. It's imperative that I get out of town right away. There are people down here who don't want me to tell you what I know.*

*Meet me by the Black Sun sculpture in Volunteer Park. I've been there before, and I know how to find it. It's very public and it's safe. I'll get there as soon as I can. I'll stay until 10:00 PM and will look for you then if not before.*

*Please hurry. These people down here are capable of anything. I'm scared.*

*Carrie's friend,*

*Candy Peterson*

Jon looked around at the people in the pressroom. The Black Sun sculpture was located across a cobblestone drive from the Seattle Asian Art Museum and right in front of the Volunteer Park reservoir. It was a large hollow disc chiseled from smooth black stone, and many in Seattle took it to represent the cold, empty space in the winter sky where the warming sun was supposed to be. It was a favorite tourist spot. Visitors standing in front of it could see the Space Needle behind the reservoir through its center. Jon hit the reply icon.

*I'll be there. Wait for me. How will I recognize you? I'm about six feet tall and have black hair. I'll arrive in a black Explorer.*

He waited for several minutes for a return e-mail.

Another reporter, Jeanne Berdik, asked Tindall if they'd found any fingerprints at the crime scene. Jon rolled his eyes. Berdik was an airhead, but he had to admit that she looked pretty good in front of a camera. She was a hottie. Tindall explained that they'd found hundreds of fingerprints in the records room, maybe thousands. It would take time to sort it all out.

Jon kept an eye on his BlackBerry. Someone asked why they didn't have more security in the hospital at night. He waited a few minutes more. Rod Bench wanted to know if the murders would affect tourism. Jon's e-mail remained unanswered. He listened for a few minutes more; then he excused himself, stood, squeezed by the reporters standing near the doorway at the back of the room, and began his long trip back to Seattle.

∷   ∷   ∷

Traffic going north on I-5 was maddeningly slow, and Jon worked his way through and around it as fast as possible. He received a warning citation from a highway patrolman for excessive lane changes at Olympia and a speeding ticket near Tacoma, where the speed limit abruptly drops to 55 MPH. He arrived at the entrance to Volunteer Park at 8:40.

He'd called Mavis along the way, asking her if she knew anything about the information Candy referred to in her e-mail. She'd said that she didn't. He'd asked her if she'd heard from Carrie. She'd said that she'd prefer not to answer that question. He drove past the old water tower at the park's entrance and parked his Explorer on the museum side of the cobblestone drive. Then he looked for a single woman somewhere in the vicinity of the Black Sun.

The area around the museum was filled with people, mostly tourists. He checked his BlackBerry; again there were no candypete messages. He got out of his car and approached several single women hanging out near the sculpture. Some welcomed his approach, some did not; none answered to the name Candy. He searched the crowd. He had no idea at all what she looked like. He mingled for a short while and then went back to his car to wait.

At 9:30 the museum doors closed and were locked. By 9:45 the temperature was starting to drop; the few people still sitting at the base of the sculpture began to move on. By 9:50 the park was relatively deserted. At 9:59 Jon again opened the front door to his car. It took him less than a minute to walk back across the cobblestone drive. The Black Sun seemingly sucked the heat out of the surrounding air; he shivered.

He watched the hands of his watch as they reached 10:00, 10:03, 10:05, and 10:10.

The lights on the top floor of the museum went out.

The hands on his watch moved to 10:15 and then to 10:30.

A reflection of the full moon shone on the reservoir.

He called Karen to tell her where he was and what had happened in Ocean City. He told her about Candy's e-mail. With Carrie Williams missing, two linked murders in two days, stolen medical records, and mysterious digital tapes, it was time to get her involved with the case. He could use her help.

"Stay warm," she said. "I'll be in the bedroom with Leon, waiting for you."

He answered, "Lucky Leon."

He again checked his watch: 10:50, then 11:00, then 11:30.

A sign near the reservoir's edge read:

## PROTECT SEATTLE'S WATER QUALITY
## DON'T FEED THE BIRDS

He stayed there until midnight, the time that the park closed. Candy Peterson was nowhere in sight.

# Chapter 12

JON CAME HOME to a darkened house. Leon greeted him at the door, and after a few wags of his tail, he wasted no time waddling out past him into the yard to fertilize the garden. Karen was waiting for him in the bedroom. She was sitting on the bed, wearing one of his white button-down shirts and not much else, reading a book. "Hi, Karen," he said as he walked over to the side of the bed. "What are you reading?" He sat down next to her.

"*Cube 6*. It's a thriller." She tossed the book down on the covers.

He picked it up and looked at it. "This stuff will rot your mind, you know." He put the book back down.

"I know; it keeps me up at night.

"It sounds like you had quite a trip." She wiggled up against her pillow and pulled her knees up under her chin. "Tell me about your mysterious rendezvous with Candy what's-her-name."

"She didn't show." He kicked off his shoes and moved over next to her against the pillow. "I hope she's all right. You should've seen her e-mail. She sounded desperate." He told her about waiting in the parking lot until midnight.

"Poor baby," she cooed. "What's the matter? Never been stood up before?" Leon began scratching at the back door, ready to come back inside.

Jon said, "I hope that's all it is." He again went over what had happened in Ocean City. "I'm afraid it might be something else."

"Let's hope not." She snuggled a little closer to him and then hooked her arm through his. "While you were waiting in the park, I did a little Carrie Williams background search of my own. This girl's not exactly all that she seems."

Jon turned towards her and lifted an eyebrow. "You used your special police-access programs?"

"That and Google. I googled her and then just followed the leads. From what I was able to find there and in our SPD database, it looks like Carrie Williams may be a troubled young woman. No doubt she's a medical superstar, and she looks just fine on the surface, but her mother was shot and killed in Pioneer Square earlier this year."

"Yes, I know that."

"Well, she really took it hard. When the police couldn't find the shooter, she went out looking for him on her own. Apparently she's a very strong-willed woman. She spent all of her free nights out on the streets questioning anyone who would talk to her. She filed for a concealed-weapon permit and got one. She became obsessed. We had complaints."

"We?"

"The police. She was warned about vigilante action and strongly advised to leave it alone. She was referred to a psychiatrist and maybe even started on antidepressants. I don't know whether she's still on the medications or not, but I know for a fact that she's still looking for the perp that shot her mother. She keeps in contact with some of the musicians that hang out in the district."

"So she's seriously screwed up?"

"She certainly was at one time; I don't know about now. By the way, do you still have Candy Peterson's e-mail? I'd like to look at it."

"Sure. I picked it up with my BlackBerry. It'll be in my mailbox under candypete@aol.com. You can use my computer. I'll go let Leon in while you check it out. Let me know what you think." Jon got up and left to open the door for Leon.

When he got back, Karen was in his office, bending over the computer on his desk. His shirt was riding up on the back of her legs, way up. He felt a familiar stirring as he walked up behind her and looked over her shoulder. "Find anything of interest in there?" He slipped his hands around her waist under the shirt. He was greeted by nothing but bare skin.

"Umm, maybe," she answered with a coy smile. "How about you? You find anything of interest in there?" She turned around in his arms.

"Umm, maybe." He reached around behind her back and shut down the computer. "It's getting late, don't you think? We can finish this later." He slowly inched his hands up her sides and started carefully unbuttoning the shirt, one button at a time, until it fell open. "Why don't we go into the bedroom?"

She batted her eyes. "Oh, how conventional!"

Jon slid the shirt off her shoulders. She stood in front of him for a few seconds and then took his hand and led the way into the bedroom. Leon followed them in. Karen quietly slipped under the sheets, waiting for Jon as he undressed.

Leon sat down by the edge of the bed. He watched as Jon slid in beside her and moved over to her side. He perked up his ears as he listened to the giggling and the rhythms of the moment. His nose wiggled as he smelled the pheromones. And when it was over, finally over, he yawned, scratched behind his ear for a moment or two, and then walked out into the kitchen to check out his food bowl. It had been a long day, and he'd seen it all before.

# Chapter 13

Seattle's drinking water comes from the Cedar River watershed, a drainage basin in the Cascade Mountains, and it has been judged by at least two independent polls to be among the very best in the country. Water aficionados have claimed that it contains just the right balance of minerals and silica to give it a crisp, bright taste. It's piped into the city through a large six-foot-diameter hundred-year-old pipe, first to a chlorination and fluorination treatment facility and then on to a system of open-air reservoirs for storage and further distribution to the neighborhoods. Although there have been complaints about the open-air nature of the reservoirs—bird droppings have been a problem—the water department regularly tests to ensure that the water is safe. As a matter of record, there haven't been any serious water-quality issues since the rupture of a secondary distribution pipe near the city's south end in 1987.

The open-air reservoir at Volunteer Park serves Seattle's Capitol Hill and Madison Park neighborhoods as well as parts of the central city. It's made of cement, is roughly triangular, and is located just to the west of the Black Sun across from the Seattle Asian Art Museum. It was constructed over a century ago after the great Seattle earthquake and fire. And although the reservoir had originally been easily accessible, visitors to the park can no longer reach its waters because of a ten-foot-high security fence. The fence, set back thirty-five feet from the water's edge, is attached to the sides of a pump house located on the reservoir's southwest corner. The only way in or out of the complex is through the pump house door.

Bruce McCaw, the foreman of a three-man maintenance crew from the city water department, was standing by his truck, talking to his crew, smoking a cheap Swisher-Sweet cigar. It was his job to continually inspect the city's water distribution system and to test the water quality. Today was his day to check on the reservoir at Volunteer Park. He was tired and hung over from a long night at the Sunset Club, not to mention that he had to work two jobs to make ends meet.

McCaw tossed his cigar, grabbed his equipment, and led his crewmen down the grass-covered hill from the Black Sun sculpture to the edge of the reservoir fence. From there they walked southwest around its periphery to the pump house door. In response to the release of the 9/11 Commission report, the chain links of the fence had been topped with barbed wire to further discourage uninvited guests from entering the facility.

McCaw unlocked the door and stepped inside. The crew was immediately greeted by the sound of cascading water as it rushed over the distribution system's open-air water gate. McCaw and his crew members moved onto the open metal grid flooring of the pump house's upper platform to survey its operation.

A series of pipes of various sizes came into the building from below and to the left of the spot where the crew was standing, and they connected to several large pumps on their right. A plaque on one of the pumps identified it as one of the original pieces of equipment installed over a century ago. A control panel with ancient-looking switches, lights, and gauges was located on the wall to their right, and a large circular hand crank attached to the water gate was also to their right. It was an emergency mechanical shutoff override to be used in case of an electrical failure. As they moved farther inside the facility, the humming sound from the pumps became audible beneath the splashing of the water.

Water was pumped into the reservoir through the incoming pipes and then released through the water gate into a gravity-based distribution system. It flowed to the neighborhoods as needed. Auxiliary pumps were available and could be used in a back-up capacity. It was an old system, but it was reliable, and simplicity was its chief asset. McCaw walked over to begin his inspection of the facility.

The first items on his checklist were the pumps, followed by the control panel. As he went to work, his crew mates went outside through a back door to check on the reservoir. They walked the inner periphery of the fence, looking for cracks in the cement and other anomalies. They searched the water for foreign bodies and took water samples for later analysis. Then they joined McCaw back inside for a thorough inspection of the water gate.

Water rushed out of the reservoir and over the top of the water gate just inside the pump house walls. From there it fell into a collection pool to be sent out through the outflow pipes. It was difficult to see anything through the foamy turbulence in the water, and it was only by luck that the crew was able to spot the pale, shimmering shape near an outflow valve. It was below the surface of the collection pool and looked like it had been partially sucked into the Capitol Hill distribution pipe. The shape was difficult to define in the burbling current. It shimmied back and forth in the flowing water, moving in and out of the pipe and in and out of view.

McCaw walked down the metal grate steps to a lower landing for a closer look. Water splashed on his clothes as he stood over and directly in front of the cascade. He peered down over the railing at the clearly visible, semi-amorphous shape. It moved in and out of focus below the surface of the water. He watched for at least a minute, and then when the bubbles briefly cleared, he shouted, "Holy shit!" He turned around to look at his crew mates. "You guys gotta come down here. You aren't going to believe this."

They rushed down the steps to take a look.

McCaw pulled out his cell phone. He pushed a speed-dial number and reported his discovery to his supervisor. They had a short conversation. "It's the Goddamnedest thing I've ever seen," he said. Then he called the police.

: : :

It was close to noon when Karen got the call. She'd just finished a workout in the gym, had taken a shower, and was eating banana yogurt for lunch in her office at the Public Safety Building when the phone rang. Her hair was still wet. She licked off her spoon and picked up the receiver.

"Detective Lieutenant Karen Able, homicide."

"Karen, it's Robbie. We've got a case." Detective Sergeant Robbie Washington worked with Karen in homicide. He was her part-time partner and always her friend. About a year ago they'd worked together on a task force to solve a well-publicized serial murder. It was her first case as a lieutenant and her first time as a task-force leader.

"What have you got?" she asked.

"We have an apparent homicide in Volunteer Park. There's a body stuck in an outflow pipe at the pump house up by the reservoir."

"A water-distribution-system outflow pipe?" She looked at the glass of water sitting next to her yogurt. She wondered which reservoir sent water to police headquarters.

"You got it. It's a woman," he said. "Her body looks like it's in one piece, but it's hard to tell for sure from our vantage point. We'll get a closer look when they shut off the water."

"Candy Peterson?" Karen immediately thought of Jon.

"Who?"

"Candy. ... Oh, never mind. It could be just a coincidence. I'll tell you about it later. Where are you now?"

"I'm in the pump house. The door was locked when a city work crew arrived here earlier this morning and discovered the body. It can only be locked from the outside."

"Has the forensic team been there yet, and what about the medical examiner?"

"I'm going to call them just as soon as we're off the phone."

"I can be there in twenty minutes," she said. "Wait for me. Don't do anything with the crime scene until I get there. I'd like first crack at it." She hung up the receiver. Then she called Jon.

:  :  :

Karen tossed the rest of her lunch into her wastebasket. She went down to the parking lot to pick up her unmarked car, flipped on its siren, and rushed over to Volunteer Park. By the time she arrived, there were already four blue-and-whites obstructing the driveway to the Asian Art Museum, one with its lights still flashing. Robbie's car was parked farther down the drive toward the Victorian greenhouse.

The crowd that had gathered near the Black Sun seemed to be growing by the minute. Two uniformed patrolmen stood between the crowd and the down slope leading from the sculpture to the reservoir. Yellow crime-scene tape marked off an area from the west side of the Black Sun down to the fence and then southwest around the periphery of the fence to the pump house. Karen could see Robbie in his tailored brown suit standing a full head taller than the others just outside the pump house door.

Removing an aluminum briefcase from her car trunk, she made her way through the crowd to the crime-scene tape. She greeted the two uniformed officers, showed them her detective shield, and moved on to join Robbie at the pump house door. Robbie ended his conversation with Bruce McCaw when he saw her approach with her evidence-collection kit.

"Hi, Karen," he said. "Quite a crowd." He nodded up toward the museum.

She smiled as she greeted him. "Yeah, and they're still coming. Everyone's got a police scanner these days. How's it going?"

"I think we've got it covered." Robbie glanced over at McCaw. "This is Bruce McCaw, the crew foreman." Karen introduced herself; McCaw extended his hand and they shook. "We got a call from the work crew at 11:14 this morning. They discovered the body while doing a routine check of the water supply system." Karen looked past the crime-scene tape into the pump house.

"Patrolman Frink arrived here about eight minutes after we

got the call. He's up by the sculpture working crowd control if you want to talk to him. He confirmed the discovery." Robbie looked at his watch to document the time of Karen's arrival, and then he continued, "He got the work crew out of the pump house, called in his report, and then cordoned off the whole area. I think he did a pretty good job. I poked around for a few minutes after I got here, and then I called you."

Karen looked back at the taped-off grassy area as it extended up toward the sculpture. "There's little chance we'll find anything back there," she said. "It's pretty well contaminated.'

"Yeah, I know. I already checked it out, but Frink had his heart in the right place. We'll take down the tape later today when we leave."

Karen kneeled down and picked up some dried earth. She watched it crumble as she rubbed it between her thumb and fingers; then she stood back up. "What's it like inside?"

"The crime scene's in pretty good shape," he said. "As far as I can determine, there've only been six people in there since the murder—the four members of the work crew, Patrolman Frink, and me. Whoever did it unlocked the door with a pick, or maybe a key, and then locked it again after he, she, or they left. Forensics should get here any time now, but I called you first, and now that you're here, I'll call the M.E. You said you wanted first crack at the crime scene."

They both looked up when she heard the telltale thwapping of an approaching helicopter. It had KIRO 7 spelled out on its side. Soon the press would be swarming all over the place.

"Let's go before that helicopter camera crew zooms in on us," she said. They ducked under the yellow crime-scene tape and walked together into the pump house. They were greeted by the sounds of rushing water frothing through the water gate.

"She's in there," Robbie said, pointing to the pool of rushing water beyond the railing. "That's how they found her."

Karen approached the rail. "That's her down there?" She saw a pale shape moving below the surface of the flowing water. "It's hard to tell that it's a body."

"That's her," Robbie said. "Arms and legs kind of move in and out of the pipe with the current. We'll get a better look after they shut off the water. They're supposed to be rerouting from the other reservoirs to Capitol Hill, and when they're finished, they'll shut it off here."

Karen stared down at the shifting pale shape as it moved from side to side with changes in the water flow. After a minute or so she put her briefcase down on the metal grate flooring, opened it, and removed several glass tubes, plastic bags, and metal scrapers. The scrapers had been sterilized in an autoclave and were wrapped in individual paper coverings. She put the items in her pockets, removed a pair of latex gloves, and put them on. Then she started to work the crime scene, beginning with the floor of the upper landing.

She started at the door, walking back and forth from one wall to the other in a grid pattern, keeping her head down and her eyes focused on the floor grate the whole time.

After finding, removing, and labeling several samples of dried mud and dirt, she said, "Robbie, look at this."

There was a small amount of what looked like dried blood near the base of the control panel. She took out a scraper, peeled off its paper wrapper, scraped off a sample, and put it in a specimen tube. Then she labeled the tube and continued her search.

"No telling how much blood fell here," she said. "Most of

it probably ran through the grate into the water. Be sure the photographer gets a picture of this."

She moved on.

Next she walked around the periphery of the upper landing, systematically looking at the walls, the control panel and the pumps, and then at the ceiling. "I can't see anything here," she said. "Maybe forensics will get us some useful prints." She walked down the steps and repeated the procedure on the lower level.

There was a knock on the outside of the door. Bruce McCaw stuck his head in and said that he could shut off the water any time they were ready. Robbie told him to wait until the photographer arrived.

A second helicopter had joined the first one in a circling hover over the reservoir—this one from KING TV. A KOMO news van pulled in behind the blue-and-white with the flashing lights. It raised its antenna as a news crew set up for an on-the-scene report. The crowd continued to grow, buzzing with the rumor of a body in the water.

The forensics team finally arrived with its photographer and followed the yellow tape down to the pump house. The photographer started to snap his photos. The team scraped more of the blood off the metal grate flooring into more glass sample tubes. Then they dusted for prints. When they finished, Robbie gave the word to shut off the water flow.

The sound of the rushing water died away. The pale body stopped its movement as the current slowed and then stopped. It was definitely a female.

It settled on its side. The head, shoulders, and left arm were wedged inside the outflow pipe. She was bare-legged, and her shoes were gone. Her blue skirt had been sucked up over her torso, obstructing the view of her upper body. She was wearing white bikini panties. If there was a purse, it had been sucked away along with her shoes. As the water level dropped, the beginnings of grayish lesions of decomposition became visible in several places on her mottled flesh. She'd been in the water at least twelve hours, probably longer. From what they could see so far, she looked to be between twenty and thirty-five years old.

The photographer snapped off another series of photos.

The water drained away.

The body settled to the bottom.

Karen instructed the others to remain where they were before pulling a flashlight out of her evidence kit and then climbing over the railing down to the level of the distribution pipe. She stood in an inch or so of water as she began to examine the body. She started with the exposed legs and then examined the arm.

"Send the photographer down here, will you?" she said. "I want some close-ups of this before I try to pull her out."

The photographer climbed down and took his close-ups. Karen then reached into the pipe and felt all around the body. It was clear on all sides. She grabbed the vic's skirt and gently pulled it back down over her legs; then she turned on her flashlight and shone it inside the pipe. "She has brown hair," she said. "Can you shoot some photos in there?"

The photographer's flash went off again and again, each time from a slightly different angle. When he was done, Karen said, "OK, I'm going to pull her out." The photographer backed off, and Karen grabbed the vic's ankles.

"Be careful with the skin," Robbie said from over the railing. "It looks like it's all puffed up and loose. You could pull it off."

"You want to do it?" She looked up at him on the metal grate, smiled a disingenuous smile, and then pulled on both legs with a firm yank. The body slid out of the pipe and onto the floor of the water gate with a flabby-sounding splat. It landed face down.

Karen kneeled to inspect the vic—first her right arm, then the back of her head, her neck, and her back. She was wearing a white blouse. There was no obvious evidence of trauma. But when she turned the body over, she saw two small holes—two gunshot entry wounds, one through the blouse in the center of her chest and the other in the middle of her forehead. There was no blood.

Karen took out her pen and gently probed the forehead wound. The edges were puckered. There were no powder burns, although the powder, if it had ever been there, would've been washed away by the flowing water. She'd have to wait on the autopsy to be sure.

She unbuttoned the vic's blouse. The bullet had gone through her bra just to the left of midline. She reached around her back, confirmed that there was no exit wound, unsnapped the bra, and gently moved it out of the way. There was a puckered entry wound through the medial edge of the left breast. It was similar to the one in her forehead. Again she probed the bloodless wound.

"She was shot through the head and the heart, a double tap, probably a low-velocity .22-caliber load," she said. "It looks professional."

The photographer continued to snap her photos.

"OK, you can send down the forensic guys," she said. "Is the medical examiner here yet?"

"She's up here behind me," Robbie answered. "She has her whole team."

"Hi, Karen." It was Dr. Cristina Cook. She stuck her head

over the railing. "What do you have down there?"

Karen stood up. "Come on down and see for yourself," she answered. Cook climbed down. Karen pointed out the entrance wounds and the beginnings of skin decomposition lesions, then described how she found the body. Then she climbed back up to the lower landing.

"Let's go outside," she said to Robbie when she reached him. They walked together to the upper landing and then out into the sunshine. Several more news vans had arrived, all of them setting up for on-the-scene reports.

"This is going to be a media circus in a few minutes," she said.

"No doubt about that." Robbie shielded his eyes from the sun as he looked up the hill toward the media vans and the sculpture.

"So what do you think so far?" Karen turned her back to the long lenses of the television cameras. "Any ideas?" They started to walk.

Robbie surveyed the gathering equipment and crowd. He scratched his chin. "As you said, it looks professional. Casual shooters go for the big guns, at least nine millimeters, more often .38s, .44s, or .45s. I think this was a professional hit. I wonder who she was."

They stopped by the edge of the reservoir. She eyed the news teams with their cameras and microphones. "Try running her prints against the nursing staff at the Sisters of Mercy Hospital in Ocean City, Oregon. It might save some time." She peeled off her latex gloves and put them in her pocket.

"The vic's prints?" Robbie questioned. "What do you know that I don't know?" One of the helicopters broke its hover and slid away out of sight behind the museum. The visuals weren't worth the price of its Jet-A fuel.

"Candy Peterson," she answered. A gust of wind, probably the tail of a helicopter downdraft, blew a cluster of leaves up in the air. They swirled around, and one landed in her hair. She brushed it away. "Jon was supposed to meet her here last night. She didn't show up. She's a nurse from Ocean City. She told him she'd meet him by the Black Sun and said that she was scared about something. It had something to do with the murders down there."

"Jon as in Jon Kirk the reporter?" Robbie asked. He furrowed his forehead.

"Uh-huh," she answered. "The one and only."

His eyes narrowed. "Karen! After all that's happened between you two, you're not still hanging around with that guy, are you?"

"Now and then," she answered.

"I'll bet it's more than just now and then." Robbie curled his lip. "He's an asshole. You should stay away from him."

"He has his good points," she countered.

"He's going to get you into trouble again. You know it and I know it. Even he knows it! Don't you ever learn?"

"OK, OK. He's an asshole, but he's my asshole. Besides, I think he loves me."

Robbie rolled his eyes. "Jon Kirk." He shook his head. "This is going to get interesting."

# Chapter 14

JON WAS AT HIS DESK in the newsroom, which was in its usual state of controlled chaos. Shouted conversations, clacking keyboards, ringing telephones, people running back and forth—the room was in perpetual motion. It felt almost alive. Jean Viereck, the paper's gossip columnist, screeched when she found out that she hadn't been invited to the mayor's sixtieth birthday party, the social event of the season. She'd have to talk with his social coordinator about that. A group of sports writers was guffawing about something a Mariners' starting pitcher had done in a sports bar. The omnidirectional cacophony of noise and confusion seemed to come from everywhere at once and nowhere in particular, but Jon was oblivious to it all. His mind had shut it out. His brain was exquisitely focused. He was working on a story.

Candy Peterson was dead. Although her identity had yet to be confirmed, he knew that it had to be her. She'd been assassinated—shot in the head and the heart. Karen said that she'd call him to confirm when they had a definitive fingerprint match.

The electronic media had reported the murder, but none of the background, and they hadn't a clue about details or motive.

Jon knew about the connection to Ocean City and to Carrie Williams. The story was his exclusive, and he was determined to explore it. What had she said in her e-mail? *It's imperative that I get out of Ocean City right away. There are people down here who don't want me to tell you what I know.* What was that all about? Whatever it was, he was now right in the middle of it, and he was making it his business to find out.

Who was Candy Peterson, who were her friends, who knew that she was coming to Seattle, and what was it that she was coming to tell him? And finally, how did it tie in to the assisted suicide and tissue-processing activities at the Sisters of Mercy Hospital?

Jon needed an expert on medical ethics. He'd called Herschel Boyd, the chairman of the Ethics Department at the University of Washington, and was on the phone with him when his intercom light flashed on. Boyd seemed like he was in a hurry. He'd been packing for a quick, unscheduled trip out of the country and was quite relieved when Jon told him that he'd have to abbreviate their conversation. Boyd said he'd be out of contact for an undetermined period of time and told Jon not to call him back. Jon broke their connection. He then pushed the intercom button and answered.

"Jon, would you come in here for a minute?" It was Chris Collins, his editor.

"Uh, sure, Chris. What's up?"

"I'll tell you when you get here. It won't take long."

"OK, I'll see you in a minute." He hung up and walked across the newsroom to his office.

Collins' office was located in a corner of the open-office-concept newsroom. It was the only closed office on the floor. Jon approached his editor's door and knocked.

"Come in!" a voice boomed from inside.

Collins was seated at his desk. His office was in its usual state of disarray. A cork bulletin board on the wall behind him had notes tacked to notes tacked to notes. Papers of various sorts littered surfaces everywhere. The only clear space was his computer stand with its computer, his connection to the paper's central nervous system. He kept it to the right of his desk, and it was always turned on.

"What is it, Chris?" Jon asked as he entered the room.

"Good job on the Candy Peterson piece," he said. "Thanks for the preview. Have a seat." He pointed to one of the chairs in front of him. Then he pressed his intercom key. "Vicki, would you ask Lizzy Carlstrom to come in here, please?" His secretary said that she would. "Thanks." Then once again addressing Jon, he asked, "You're sure about the victim's identity? She hasn't been officially ID'd by the police."

"We'll know soon enough," he answered. "Karen said she'd call as soon as the ID's confirmed."

"Your policeman friend?"

"That's right. It shouldn't take long to run the prints."

"Let's hope not. I'd like to get this thing into print."

There was a knock on the door. "Come in." Liz Carlstrom entered the office. She was holding a packet of papers in her hand. "Sit over there." Collins pointed at a chair next to Jon. She sat. Then he cleared his throat. "Jon, I want you to turn the Candy Peterson story over to Lizzy."

"What?" Jon rose up off his seat. Lizzy looked less than surprised.

"Sit down," Collins said to Jon.

"But ..."

"Sit down." Jon glanced over at Lizzy, and then he slowly sat. "You're too close to it," Collins continued. "You're the reason Peterson came to Seattle. You can't write your own story. There's no objectivity; it's against the rules." He turned to Liz. "Lizzy, Jon will give you what he's done so far. You take it from there."

"Like hell I will," Jon said.

"Like hell you won't," Collins answered. "Bitch and moan all you want, but you'll do it. You'll do it because deep down you know it's the right thing to do. Now let's cut the crap, shall we? Lizzy gets the Candy Peterson part of the story; you keep the rest. That's it. Now both of you get out of here and go to work."

Jon started to say something. Collins glared at him. "Yes?"

"Uh ..."

Lizzy waved the packet of papers she held in her hand. "Oh, yeah," Collins said. "Give those to Jon." Then he reached into his desk, pulled out a Tootsie Pop, unwrapped it, and jammed it into his mouth. He'd been trying to quit smoking for years. "I don't want to hear anything more about this." The Tootsie Pop bounced up and down when he talked. "Now go." Lizzy and Jon got up, looked at each other, and then left the room.

: : :

Karen sat in her smallish office in the Seattle Public Safety Building, her feet up on her desk. Her desk was neat. Her room was functional. Her only personal touch, a silver-framed photograph of her father wearing Vietnam-era jungle fatigues and a green beret, was on a file cabinet to her right. Robbie had just walked in the door.

"You were right about the vic," Robbie said. "She's been

identified as Candy Peterson, a nurse from Ocean City, Oregon.

"Fingerprints?" Karen asked.

"Nope. Her fingers were all swollen from her time in the water, and we couldn't get good prints."

"Dental records?"

"Breast implants. They took the serial numbers off her breast implants and matched them with the manufacturer's product registry. It's a new one on me. They're still doing the autopsy."

"It must be a slow day in the M.E.'s office," she said. "They usually keep their patients on ice for a while before they operate." Karen swung her feet off her desk and onto the floor.

Robbie sat down in one of the two chairs facing her desk and pushed the other one aside with his foot. "They already got the bullets out. They were twenty-twos, just as you thought—hollow points, one from her brain and one from her chest. From what I heard, they really ripped her up inside, put a big hole in her heart, and turned half of her brain into mush. They flattened and fragmented when they hit."

"No wonder there weren't any exit wounds."

"As you said, it looks professional. I think we're dealing with hired guns."

Karen pushed some papers to the side of her desk. "Anything else?"

"Yeah, and you're going to love this part. All of her fingers were broken, all ten of them, each one snapped in a different place. Actually they weren't just snapped; the bones were crushed. They were mutilated. They must have pinned her against the floor grate and smashed them one at a time."

Karen sat up in her chair. "She was tortured?"

"That's the way I see it." Robbie scratched the five o'clock shadow growing on his chin. "Somebody was after something, something important, something worth hiring a professional to get. And I don't think they got whatever it was that they wanted, either, not with all ten of her fingers broken. They'd have stopped if they'd got what they wanted. These guys were professionals. They'd have ended it and killed her." Robbie slowly looked up toward the ceiling. He scanned across as if he were counting acoustic tiles. "Maybe it's time we had a talk with your boyfriend." His eyes slid back down to hers. "Jon was her only known connection to Seattle, wasn't he? I'd like to hear what he has to say about all of this." When she didn't answer right away, he added, "You did say that the vic came to Seattle specifically to see him, didn't you?" His eyes fixed onto hers.

"I'll talk to Jon," she answered. "I'll take care of it. I don't think he knows anything more than I've already told you. Carrie Williams is the one we really need to find and interview."

"You're sure?" Robbie persisted. "Any little bit of information Jon has could be important."

She stared back at him. "I said I'd take care of it. And while I'm doing that, you can check the bullets with ballistics, see if we can get a computer match. Maybe the shooter used this gun before."

"OK, but do you really think that's such a good idea? About Kirk, I mean. He's not a suspect, but he's our only living direct contact. We need to know what he knows. And as far as objectivity is concerned ..." He waited for a response. There was none forthcoming. "Maybe it would be better if I talked with him. It's cleaner that way. No entanglements. I'll ask him to come down to an interrogation room. You can watch through the mirror if you want."

"That won't be necessary," she said. "I said I'd take care of this."

Robbie broke his stare and looked away. "Whatever you say."

"About the slugs, they're too fragmented and deformed for computer analysis. And we don't have any casings. Best guess is that the shooter used a revolver. A pro wouldn't risk losing an ejected shell from an automatic, especially with the floor grate in the pump house the way it is. The CSI unit went over the place in detail, and they didn't find a thing."

"What about the samples I gave them?"

"Not done yet. They'll get back to us with their preliminary site analysis tomorrow. They took a lot of material from the body, along with the soil, blood, and fiber samples from the floor. They also have a lot of prints to sift through."

"Let me know as soon as you hear anything."

Robbie stood up. He moved over to the window and watched as a ferry made its way across Puget Sound toward Bainbridge Island. Seagulls were following close alongside the open passenger decks, hoping for a handout. Every now and then a group of them would swoop down and fight over a bit of food that had been tossed in their direction. He could almost hear their screeches.

"About Jon ..."

"Robbie," Karen interrupted, "I'll talk to him tonight." Robbie turned from the window to directly face her. "I'll talk to Jon. If he has anything pertinent to say, I'll set up a formal interview for tomorrow. You can do it. OK?" She paused for a moment. "Is that OK?"

Robbie answered, "OK, I guess."

"And, Robbie, I won't be on the other side of the mirror."

"Sure, Karen," he answered. "As I said, whatever you say."

# Chapter 15

Jon left work early. He knew that Collins was right about being too close to the story, but that didn't seem to help. He was pissed. He hated to lose an exclusive. He gave Lizzy his material and then left the newsroom to work at home. He was at his desk in his converted spare bedroom when he opened her packet of information.

It was material for a news story. Somebody had invented a replacement for the venerable star valve, the valve used in most commercial toilets around the world. The inventor, John Runstad, an engineer who lived on a houseboat on Lake Union, was tired of having his toilet overflow every time he stressed it with a capacity load. The revolutionary new valve, with its improved flow dynamics, which he termed The Runstad Valve, was supposed to fix all that. It had been widely acclaimed throughout the industry.

"This is what I get in place of the Peterson story?"

Jon knew that Thomas Crapper had invented the star valve, and with it the modern toilet. He was reputedly knighted for his achievement. Would John Runstad's name become as closely associated with the device as had Crapper's? Would he be recognized in some similar fashion for his contribution? At some time in the future, would someone want to take a Runstad?

*Don't go there, Jon,* he thought to himself. This was just Collins' idea of payback for the trouble he'd caused him with the suicide tourism thing. He canned the Runstad article, tossed the papers Lizzy had given him into the wastebasket, turned his computer on, and then went to work on the Carrie Williams story. He didn't hear Karen when she opened the back door.

"Jon, are you in there?" she said as she entered the kitchen.

"I'm back here," he answered. "In the office."

"We identified the body." She walked up the three stairs into the back hallway. "No surprise. It was Candy Peterson." She continued on through the open office door. Leon followed close behind. "We identified her through her breast implants." She walked up behind him and told him about the problem with her fingerprints.

"Oh, great, an even better story. I can't wait to pass that one on to Lizzy." He was sitting at his desk looking at the screen of his Apple MacBook Pro.

"Lizzy?" Karen asked. Jon told her about Collins taking his story away. "He's right, you know," she said after he finished. "You're much too close to it. This thing looks professional." She told him about the .22-caliber low-velocity hollow points and then about the torture.

Jon spun around in his chair. "Good God!"

"All ten of her fingers were broken. It happened in the pump house. Blood on the floor grate matches her blood type. We're running a DNA analysis just to be sure.

"The way I see it," she continued, "someone found out about the meeting she'd scheduled with you in the park. They knew she had sensitive information concerning Carrie Williams and Stewart Wolf. They wanted it, whatever it was, and they didn't want you to have it. So they grabbed her, took her to the pump house, tortured her to get it, and then killed her and dumped her body over the railing into the water gate. That, or there was something that she possessed that they wanted, and they tortured her to get it before she could give it to you. Either way, the cement pump house walls and the rushing water would've masked her screams." Jon's computer timed out and put itself to sleep. Its screen went blank. He had it set to its power conservation mode.

"We found her car around the corner in the lot by the park's greenhouse. I'm really worried. This thing is getting out of control."

"Yeah, me, too," Jon said. "Does anybody else know about this? I mean, anybody else in the media?" His face became animated.

"Jon, you don't get it, do you? Can't you think of anything besides your story? You don't understand. You're in danger here. I'm not worried about the case. I'm worried about you. Whoever killed Candy is going to want to know what she told you, what she e-mailed you. That's part of what they tortured her to get. They're going to want to know just exactly what and how much you know."

"Let's not get too melodramatic here," Jon answered. "She didn't tell me anything."

"So you say, but they don't know that. You're going to have to watch yourself. You need to be careful." Jon thought a moment and then looked down at his fingers.

"Jon, you *have* told me everything, haven't you?" Karen searched his eyes. "You're the reason the vic came to Seattle. You're the connection between Candy, Carrie Williams, and

Stewart Wolf." She moved in a little closer. "I can't afford to have you hold out on me. It's important that you tell me everything. No surprises. You have to be honest with me."

"No surprises," Jon answered. "I promise. You already know everything I know." He started to fidget just a bit.

Karen continued her lock on his eyes. "That's good, because Robbie's concerned."

"Robbie?" Jon broke eye contact. "Of course. Your overprotective partner. Well, you can tell him for me to mind his own business."

Karen pulled back and replied, "This is his business." Then she smiled. "But I'll tell him that we talked and that there's nothing to be concerned about." She paused and then added, "Jon? There isn't anything to be concerned about, is there?"

"NO, KAREN! THERE'S NOTHING TO BE CONCERNED ABOUT!"

"Good."

"Fine." He turned back around to face his computer. "Don't talk to any other reporters about this, OK?"

"Am I sleeping with any other reporters?"

"I should hope not!"

"Then don't worry." She reached over his shoulder, gently brushing against him as she moved and tapped his computer keyboard; his computer woke up to his favorite screensaver, an image of Karen sitting by a mountain lake in her hiking shorts. "I remember that hike," she said, "a seventeen-miler. It took us all day to get up there. It was cold that night, even in our sleeping bags." She tapped the keyboard again, and a data file came up. "What are you working on?"

"I've been doing a little research," he said. "And while I was trying to connect the dots between Carrie Williams and Stewart Wolf, it occurred to me that I've been going about this thing the wrong way. I've spent way too much time on Carrie Williams and not enough time on Stewart Wolf. There are several Stewart Wolfs in Oregon, but none from Ocean City, and none of them is the Stewart Wolf who died in the Sisters of Mercy hospital. I need to find out who this guy was, and so far I haven't had much luck. There's nothing much about him in the usual search engines."

"Move over," Karen said. "Maybe you don't know where to look." Jon got out of his chair and Karen sat down. Leon moved next to her and started licking her ankles. He knew that she loved to have her ankles licked. Jon knew it, too.

Karen typed something and logged on to a restricted police site, and then she sat there for at least forty-five seconds, waiting for the system to connect. "When are you going to wire this house and get broadband?" she asked. "This dial-up connection of yours sucks! And while you're at it, you should get an Air Port."

"Didn't your mother ever teach you that patience is a virtue?"

"Yeah, yeah, yeah."

An image came up on the screen. "What are you doing?"

"Just watch." She clicked a few keys and scrolled through some data. "There he is. See, he has a Social Security number, a driver's license, credit cards." She tapped a few more keys. "A bank account ... That's interesting. Look at this." She stopped scrolling for a moment. "He has almost nineteen thousand dollars in his savings account and a little more than eight thousand dollars in his checking account, but the accounts are in his name alone. I wonder where his wife keeps her money." She quickly typed in another command. "You did say he was married, didn't you?"

"That was Carrie's story. She'd said that she'd met with her, or at least that she'd met with someone who claimed to be her. The hospital administrator, Alex Morse, said otherwise. She said he didn't have a wife."

"Let's see," Karen said. "No other bank accounts, no brokerage accounts, no life insurance, no house payments." She tapped the advance key. "He had a great credit rating. I wish I had one like that." She scrolled down the screen. "He had a job, made good money, and on the surface his bank accounts match his income."

"You can get all of that information at one site?"

"I can; it's courtesy of the Patriot Act. Scary, isn't it?" She glanced away from the screen and flashed a wily smile in Jon's direction. "Be careful, Jon. Big Brother's watching."

"Maybe it's Big Sister."

"Let's hear it for the Total Information Awareness Program." She turned and typed in another command.

"He has a birth certificate. Born in 1961." She moved the cursor and clicked on a link. It took a few seconds for the dial-up modem to transmit the connection. "He pays his taxes." She scanned through the tax data. That took a minute or two. Then all of a sudden she furrowed her brow. Her eyes narrowed.

"What's the matter?" Jon asked.

"I'm not sure." She scrolled back up. "This can't be right." She searched the site.

"What's the problem?"

"There're only four years of income tax reports in here," she said. "Just a minute." She went back to an earlier screen. Again it took awhile for the modem to connect. "This says he bought his house four years ago; he never had a mortgage. He must've paid cash."

"Maybe Big Sibling only looks back four years. I toss out my old tax records after only three."

"Not a chance," Karen answered. "Hold on." She typed a few keystrokes, searched the screen, typed a few more, and then repeated the process. It took her several minutes to search through the entire site. "This guy came to Ocean City four years ago," she said. "He opened a bank account, got some credit cards, bought a house, paid his taxes."

"A regular model citizen."

"Yeah, a model citizen, but there's a problem. Supposedly he was born in 1961, but there's nothing in here about a high school; no college." She shook her head, tapped a few keys, paused a moment, then shook her head again. "Nothing at all until four years ago. Prior to four years ago, this guy didn't exist." She took her hands off the keyboard and looked up at Jon. "This guy isn't real."

"A stolen identity?" Jon grabbed another chair, pulled it over next to Karen, and sat down. "I know how this works." He positioned the chair so that he could see the computer screen. "Check to see if a Stewart Wolf born in 1961 died at an early age. Does your Big Brother site tell you that?" Karen started to type. "The way you steal an identity is to find someone who was born within a few years of your own birth date, someone who died at an early age, and then you appropriate their birth certificate. Once you have that, credit cards, a driver's license, and the rest are easy. A new Social Security card is no problem at all." They waited for the computer's slow internal modem to connect.

"OK, here it is," she said. "Our Stewart Wolf was born in Omaha, Nebraska, in 1961. He was delivered at Clarkson Hospital at 7:51 PM." She tapped a few more keys, waited forty-five seconds or so, and then scrolled down through more data points. "And," she said as she scrolled, then paused for a moment and looked over her right shoulder at Jon, "he's still alive. There's no death certificate for the Stewart Wolf born in 1961. Nice try."

"And there are no other Stewart Wolfs that fit the bill?"

"Not that I can find."

"You're sure."

"Afraid so. Big Brother never lies." She typed in a command to shut down the computer.

"Then I guess that's it," he said. "Well, it would've made a hell of a story." He stood up and pulled his chair away. "Want to go get something to eat? I'm starved." Leon stood up when he heard the reference to food. He rarely passed on an opportunity to eat.

"A recorded birth certificate in 1961 and then nothing until four years ago?" She was staring at a blank computer screen. She thought a moment more. "There's another possibility, you know," she said. She looked away from the screen and then closed the lid to the laptop. "But we'll never find it, not in here." She stood up, stretched a little, and then looked out the window. A squirrel was sitting on the side of Jon's hot tub, eating something or other. He was dropping pieces of whatever it was all over its insulated cover. "As a matter of fact, it would be difficult to find it anywhere. I'm not even sure we *should* find it."

"What are you talking about?" Jon moved over and put his hand on her shoulder. She turned around in his chair to face him. "What's this thing that we can't find out about?"

She looked up at him for a moment. "Witness security," she said. "The federal Witness Protection Program. Maybe Stewart Wolf, or whatever his real name was, was a rat."

# Chapter 16

CARRIE PACKED THE REST of her few remaining belongings. She checked around the motel room to make sure that she hadn't left anything behind. The room was clean. There were her fingerprints, of course, and she was sure that forensic experts would be able to find traces of her DNA if they really searched, but by the time any of that could be done, she'd be long out of there. She figured that once she was out of town, none of that would matter anyway. This would be only an early waypoint on a trail that would be increasingly difficult to follow.

She finished packing and then checked her appearance in the bathroom mirror. She'd dressed in jeans and a faded Seattle Mariners sweatshirt over a white blouse, and she had a scarf tied around her head, bandana fashion, to hide her hair. She stuffed a towel under her sweatshirt to make her look heavier, and she put on some dark sunglasses to hide her eyes. It wasn't a perfect disguise, but she doubted that she'd be recognized by anyone who hadn't previously known her. She wished her face hadn't been all over the TV. Finally she adjusted the hidden towel, secured it with her belt, nodded to her reflection, and said, "Just remember what we're trying to do here." Then she glanced back at the confines of her motel room for the last time and walked out into the sunlight.

Her old friend, Chester Dorsey, had advised her to be careful and to use her head. She'd try to do both. He'd told her to come to Seattle and to sneak into his apartment the same way that she had when she was a child. Together they'd solve her problems one way or another.

She arranged to have the motel's shuttle service drive her to Hillsboro's Twin Oaks Airpark. Hillsboro was a small town just to the south and west of Portland, and Twin Oaks Airpark was a general aviation airport that catered primarily to private pilots and charter air services. It was about thirty miles away, and she paid her shuttle driver with cash. She figured that the small airport was less likely to be monitored than the terminals at Portland International. At one point she'd considered renting a car, or even buying one, but had finally decided on a charter flight as the safest way to go. It was one of the few remaining modes of travel that didn't require her to show a personal ID.

Carrie had arranged for her flight to take her to Seattle's Boeing Field and had been promised that her single-engine Cessna would be fueled and ready to go by the time she arrived. Again she figured that it was less likely to be monitored than Seattle's primary airport, Sea-Tac International. She boarded the motel's shuttle van and carefully checked the motel parking lot and surrounding area as it pulled away. The lot was nearly empty. No one followed. At one point she identified a gray Toyota several cars back that seemed to keep a consistent interval and to turn when they turned, but eventually it veered to the left at a fork in the road after they'd veered to the right, and it didn't return. She kept looking but saw nothing else.

After they arrived at the airport, she identified herself as Susan Adkins and paid for her charter flight to Seattle with cash. She was introduced to a pilot who escorted her through the field access door and onto the tarmac. He directed her to the plane, helped her climb inside, stowed her suitcase, secured her door, and taxied to the runway. Then he pushed the throttles forward and took off to start their hour-and-fifteen-minute flight north. The drone of the six-cylinder engine lulled her into a sleeplike state as they traversed the green forests of the Cascades, and she semi-slept until she was jolted awake by a hard touchdown on Boeing Field's runway 31 Left.

"We're here," said the pilot as he taxied toward the Clay Lacey Aviation terminal. "Time to move on."

Carrie looked around at the other planes on the tarmac. *Indeed it is*, she thought to herself. *It definitely is time to move on.*

# Chapter 17

The big man opened his cell phone. He moved quickly. He'd been anticipating this moment for some time. He half-smiled as he punched in his partner's number.

Her phone rang, and after she answered, he said without pause, "Our snitch at the airport called. She's here. She landed at Boeing Field in a chartered Cessna approximately fifteen minutes ago. She just left in a cab. We've got her." He walked over to his rented Buick and switched his phone to his left hand so that he could open the door.

A female voice asked him, "You're sure it's her?"

"It has to be. A six-foot-tall black woman chartering in from a backwater airport in Oregon, traveling by herself—it couldn't be anyone else. Our lineman just earned the second half of his money." He climbed inside his car and started the engine. "She chartered under the name Susan Adkins."

"Susan Adkins. I'll watch out for that name."

He released his brake, shifted into drive, and slid out into the flow of traffic. "I should be there in ten minutes, fifteen at the most. If she gets there before I do, don't wait around for me. Take care of the problem yourself. And keep a sharp lookout. She knows the city; we don't. This isn't like Miami. Find a place out front where you can watch the door. Stay out of sight, and don't let her get inside. We don't want to drag her down the stairs. We need to get this over with."

"No sweat," she answered. "Anything else?"

"Just be careful, and watch out for the cops. Half the world's looking for her. We don't want to attract a crowd."

"I'm always careful," she said. "You know that."

"Right. Don't let her or anyone else spot you."

"She'll never see a thing. Chill, will ya?"

"OK, sure, consider me chilled. I'm five minutes away from the square. I'll see you out front in ten. We'll nab her before she goes in. Things could get complicated if she gets inside, and we don't need complications."

"I'll be there."

He closed the lid on his phone and broke the connection.

# Chapter 18

OCCIDENTAL PARK in Seattle's Pioneer Square was a landmark on the original Skid Road, a term that originated in the 1800s. It was inspired by the process of sliding timber down Yesler Way to a steam-powered sawmill on the waterfront. Gold prospectors converged on the area on their way to the Yukon during the wild days of the Great Klondike Gold Rush, and gawkers came to stare at the construction of the Smith Tower, then the tallest building west of the Mississippi. An iron pergola was erected in the park to commemorate the site. It had always been a good place to lose oneself and blend in with the crowds, and Carrie was doing her best to blend in.

After landing at Boeing Field, Carrie took a cab into the city. She rode past the shadowed canyons of the old warehouse district on her way to Pioneer Square and the Elliot Bay Bookstore. The bookstore was a popular destination for both locals and tourists, and, most important for Carrie, it was always crowded. She'd left her suitcase with the receptionist at Clay Lacey Aviation.

Carrie stood on the corner by the entrance for a few minutes to make sure that she hadn't been followed, and then she ducked into a coffee shop just a few doors up the street. She identified the rear exit just in case she might need it, bought a cappuccino, sat at a table near a window, and watched the crowd outside.

She sipped her coffee.

She searched their faces.

She watched them move, searching for threats.

She checked her watch. Chester would probably be home. He usually spent his afternoons at home before leaving for dinner at Luigi's. He'd told her that when she came to Seattle, she should come to his apartment the same way that she had when she was a child, and she knew what that meant. She finished her coffee, checked the street one more time, and left for Chester's place.

Carrie walked north with the crowd. She kept a constant watch as she passed the antique shops and art galleries on First Avenue. The hairs on the back of her neck sounded an alert whenever she saw a face more than once or whenever someone spent too much time looking in her direction. The streets were crowded, and everything was in motion. By the time she reached the pergola, she was in the midst of the afternoon tourist flow.

She felt a tap on her shoulder.

Her heart thumped.

"Excuse me, miss; do you have the time? My watch stopped. I'm signed up for the underground tour, and I don't want to miss it."

It was a sailor from the *USS Nimitz*. She gave him the time.

Her heart returned to its regular rhythm.

She moved on past Cherry Street, circling around toward the alleyway behind Chester's building.

The hairs on the back of her neck returned to their standby position.

:   :   :

Chester Dorsey lived on the fourth floor of an 1890s-vintage six-story brick building. It was classic Pioneer Square, and it was in need of some repair. He lived at the back near the fire escape. The Sunset Club was on the first floor in the front, Luigi's restaurant was in the basement, and the Seattle Mystery Bookshop was up the hill across the street. The main entryway to the building, the way to the upper-floor apartments, was located adjacent to the entryway to the Sunset Club. The building was owned by Jairus Stratton, a landlord known around town as the slumlord mogul of Pioneer Square.

Two pairs of eyes watched the entrance from separate locations. Carrie approached the building as she had as a child. She circled around to the alley and found the fire escape on the back.

Carrie looked both ways, up and down the alley. It was littered with papers and smelled of urine, but she appeared to be alone. There was a dumpster about twenty yards in front of her. She walked over to the fire escape, reached up to pull down the ladder, checked the alley one more time, pulled the ladder down, and then started to climb. As a child she'd had to pull a garbage can over to reach the ladder.

She climbed up the ladder to the first metal grate landing and then moved on up the steps to the fourth floor. She could see Chester's kitchen through one of the building's large old-fashioned wooden-frame windows. The window glass was grimy, but the kitchen was just as she remembered it. It was small and clean, with a few cabinets, a refrigerator, and a four-cook-top electric combination stove and oven. No one seemed to be home.

Carrie tapped on the glass. She waited. No one came. She

tapped again, louder this time, and when again there was no response, she slipped her fingers in against the upper portion of the lower sill and pushed. The window slid open just like it always did. She curled her hands through the opening, pushing it up all the way. Then she stuck her head inside.

"Chester?"

She waited. No answer.

She took a deep breath and stepped through the window into the kitchen. Her feet made a scraping sound on the linoleum floor.

"Chester?" She looked around. There was fruit in the fruit bowl. The sink was empty and dry. The cupboards were all closed. "Chester, are you there?"

No answer.

She ran her finger over the small kitchen table. No dust. She checked out the floor. No footprints or mud. She pushed open the swinging door to the living room and the rest of the apartment. She stepped through.

"Chester?"

Chester was sitting in his favorite rocking chair with his back toward the kitchen door. The chair was still. Duct tape was wound through the wooden slats and around his chest. She started to say something but then stifled it by quickly putting a hand over her mouth. Her mind screamed, *Oh, my God!* Her voice was mute. Her lips went dry. She took a few steps forward and then to the side.

Chester's arms and wrists were taped to the arms of the rocker. His ankles were taped to the legs. His feet were bare. His chest was taped to the back of the chair, and there was a loop of tape running from the chair back around his neck. He had a strip of tape over his mouth. His fingers were bent backwards, twisted and broken, fixed at odd angles by the early stages of rigor mortis. There was a single small bullet hole in his forehead surrounded by skin puckering and a small amount of blood. A much larger bloodstain surrounded a hole in the center of his shirt and extended all the way down onto his pants.

His eyes were open and his mouth was gaping. His face was contorted. He looked as if he were still in mid-scream. There was no need for Carrie to feel for a pulse.

*Oh, Chester, I'm so sorry. I'm so sorry.*

:   :   :

The watcher across the street took his cell phone out of his pocket and called his partner. "Have you seen any sign of her?"

"Nothing yet," she answered. "How about you?"

"Nothing."

"Maybe she's not coming."

"She'll come," he said. "We just need to be patient, that's all." He scanned both ways, up and down the street.

She too scanned the street. "Maybe she went somewhere else."

"Not a chance. We have that cell phone intercept, her only known contact. And Dorsey told us that she'd show up sooner or later. There's no way he'd lie, not after all we did to him. She'll show."

The other one took a pack of cigarettes out of her pocket, shook it, and pulled one out with her lips. "Maybe there's another way in?" Her cigarette bounced up and down in her lips as she asked the question. She used an old Zippo lighter to light it.

"This is the only door. You know that."

She took a drag on her cigarette. "I think I should go up and check, just to be sure." She exhaled the smoke as she spoke.

"OK, sure, if you say so. Don't take too long."

"I'll be right back." She closed her cell phone and put it back in her pocket. Then she flicked her cigarette onto the pavement, stepped on it, and started across the street toward the entrance to the building.

The man on the corner of Cherry and First continued to watch.

: : :

Carrie closed her eyes hard and then turned away. There was nothing she could do for Chester now. She'd never meant for him to get hurt. She'd just needed a little help. It was all her fault. She felt an incredible guilt. She reached out to gently touch him on his cheek with the back of her hand, and then she heard a rattling in the front door keyhole.

Click.

Her breath stopped in mid-inspiration. Her head snapped to the left. Her pulse accelerated, then raced. She forced herself to take a short, shallow breath, and then she held it. She stood perfectly still. Her eyes were fixed on the door. The doorknob started to turn.

Adrenaline surged. Fight-or-flight reflexes took over. She bolted. She charged through the living room, banged through the swinging kitchen door, and piled out through the window. She hit the fire escape landing and then ran and slid down the stairs almost in a free fall. She was at least halfway down before the person behind her started through the window in pursuit, cell phone in hand.

"She's here," her pursuer said into the phone. "She's on the fire escape, on her way to the alley." She started down after her.

"Which way down the alley?"

"I'm not ..." She slipped on a step, and in an effort to stop her fall, she involuntarily reached for the railing while holding her phone. The impact with the railing knocked the phone from her hand, bouncing it onto the metal steps and then onto the cement below.

"Shit!" She increased her speed down the steps. By this time Carrie was sliding down the ladder onto the pavement ahead of her.

Carrie didn't take the time to look back. She ran down the alley toward First Avenue, sliced through the crowd on the sidewalk, and ran through the traffic on the street. Cars swerved and brakes squealed as she careened across. The crowd was thinner on the other side, and she was able to catch a glimpse of the person chasing her as she ran up the gentle hill toward Columbia. Then she turned the corner onto Columbia and blindly crashed into a panhandler and his cardboard sign. She almost fell, caught her balance, spun around, pushed him out of the way, and sprinted down the hill toward the waterfront. Adrenaline had taken charge. As she crossed Western and then veered right under the viaduct, she had a sense that she was increasing the distance between them. She was the faster of the two, and she was feeling like she just might get out of this mess. Then her pursuer's partner exploded out of the paper-littered shadows under the viaduct behind her. He must have circled around to try to cut her off. He was little more than half a block away, and he was closing fast.

Carrie had to do something. She had to make a choice. She wasn't going to win this race.

She swerved to her left, dodged traffic crossing Alaskan Way, cut through the line of cars coming from the Bremerton Ferry, and ran toward the ferry terminal. The man behind her had the angle on her now, and she would have to use every bit of her speed and agility if she had any chance at all of beating him to the entrance.

She didn't look back; she didn't look to the side; she didn't look anywhere at all except at the entrance. She focused hard on the entrance, and she just ran. She ran with everything she had. And by the time she'd run up the stairs in the terminal, pushed through the crowd of people buying tickets, and crashed by the ticket booth onto the gangplank loading the boat, the footsteps that she'd so keenly felt closing in behind her had been lost in the mêlée.

Carrie crossed onto the ferry, jinked to her right, and for a moment hid among the mass of passengers working their way up from the automobile decks to the coffee shop. Her lungs were burning, and she wanted to stop, but she knew she couldn't. She moved on, breathing hard, working her way against the flow of passengers down the stairs to the lower decks.

Brewster Bede, the gate security guard, had just finished his sandwich and was unscrewing the top of his coffee thermos when Carrie came crashing through the gate.

"What the …?" He spilled the coffee all over himself.

He jumped up, dropped the thermos onto the floor, and ran out of his security station behind the ticket booth into the flow of pedestrian traffic, yelling "STOP! COME BACK HERE!" and reaching for his walkie-talkie. But before he could push the push-to-talk button to alert the Washington State patrolmen stationed on the car decks, a second person, this time a man, tried to crash by the same ticket booth. He wasn't about to let that happen.

"HEY!" Bede stood tall and blocked his way. "Just what do you think you're doing?" Bede stiff-armed him in the chest. He moved to his left, continuing to obstruct the gangplank as the man tried to push around him. Bede put his hand on the spray can of Mace attached to his utility belt. "Get back in line. If you want to get on this boat, you're going to have to buy a ticket like everyone else."

The man looked down at him. He was much bigger than Bede, who was a pudgy five foot eight. The man started to say something and then thought better of it. Finally he turned and walked to the back of the ticket line. He was swearing under his breath. His partner, winded, came jogging up behind him.

"Is she on the boat?" she asked, panting as she spoke.

"Yeah." He turned his head and glared at the security guard. Bede glared back; he was talking on his walkie-talkie. "She's not going anywhere," he answered, "The boat should leave any minute now. We've got about forty-five minutes to find her before it lands."

Bede told the highway patrol that a passenger had crashed her way onto the ferry. He gave them her description. They would start a search.

The highway patrolmen started on the lower automobile deck, looking between and among the large trucks parked in the four center lanes of the super ferry. Cars were still loading onto the outer car lanes on both the main and upper car decks, and passengers were still in the process of leaving their cars for the passenger areas, coffee shop, and observation decks above.

Ferry workers were placing chocks in front of the tires of the most forward vehicles to keep them from rolling forward once the ferry was under way.

After checking to make sure the loading gangplanks were clear, Carrie's two pursuers started their search on the upper observation deck. They started at the rear end of the boat and worked their way forward, working in tandem down the two side aisles toward the front. It was easy searching the crowd. Carrie's distinctive height would make it difficult for her to blend in. When they finished with the observation deck, they moved down to the main passenger deck one floor below.

The highway patrol officers completed their search of the lower automobile deck and moved up to the car-only deck while Carrie's pursuers were systematically working their way down through the main passenger deck. Carrie was stuck in between. She'd rushed onto the boat, run down the stairs to the lower deck, seen the highway patrolmen as they began their search, darted over to the elevator, and repeatedly pushed the call button with her finger while waiting for the doors to open.

"Come on, come on! Open up!"

When the elevator came, she jumped inside, pushed "3" on the floor selection panel, and flattened herself against the side wall until the doors closed again; then she pulled the red STOP button to stop the elevator car. She was the only person in the elevator.

The alarm sounded.

RING!

She jabbed it back in. The alarm stopped. She rode up to the third deck.

The doors opened.

Nobody was waiting. Nobody got in. She stayed in the elevator. She held her breath.

The doors closed.

The elevator car didn't move.

She waited. She exhaled. Nothing happened for several minutes; then the elevator car started down. It went all the way back down to deck one.

Carrie took a deep breath. The doors opened again, this time to reveal a small group of people waiting to get in. She got out of the elevator and pushed through the grouping of passengers on her way to the line of parked cars on the port side of the boat. She looked up and down the length of cars and could see no evidence of either her pursuers or the highway patrol. The last of the cars had been parked and chocked, and ferry workers were stretching the three-foot-tall retaining fence across the open ends of the car deck.

Carrie felt the engines change pitch. Dockside gears groaned as the steel drive-on gangplank was raised about eighteen inches off the rear of the deck. Seawater behind the boat started to churn. The boat started to move. And Carrie started to run.

Carrie ran out from between the cars toward the receding dock. She ran in a total anaerobic sprint—nothing held back, nothing left in reserve. She vaulted the retaining fence in stride as if it weren't there. Dockworkers waved their hands. Ferry workers yelled for her to stop. She didn't see or hear any of it. All she saw was the widening gap between the boat and the dock. She leapt from the rear of the boat to the raised steel gangplank, made it by several feet, and kept on running. She ran past the cars starting to line up for the next ferry, and then by the tollbooth. She darted across the sidewalk, slowed only slightly as she crossed through oncoming traffic on Alaskan Way, and accelerated again. She sliced through a line of parked cars and then ran toward the debris-filled corridor beneath the Alaskan Way viaduct. A group of grimy winos watched her from the shadows as she decelerated while approaching a cement support pillar for the roadway above. Then she stopped, grabbed her abdomen, and bent over. She was totally spent. Breathing hard, she inched her way around to the back and behind the pillar. Finally she did what many of the winos had already done earlier in the day. She put her head down between her knees and threw up.

# Chapter 19

ADRENALINE IS AMAZING stuff. It can focus the body like nothing else. It can sharpen the mind to a scalpel's edge. It can obliterate pain, and it can double, sometimes even triple muscular performance. There are stories of ordinary men exhibiting extraordinary strength, summoning the ability to lift cars off trapped accident victims and the like. And there are stories of athletes exhibiting skills that on occasion seemingly defy the laws of physics and nature. But an adrenaline rush is a fleeting thing; it doesn't last. And when the adrenal glands are finished and the adrenaline is gone, you're left with nothing.

Carrie just lay there; she barely moved. She hid in the littered shadows under the viaduct for at least an hour, maybe two, maybe even more. Several ferries had come and gone; she wasn't sure how many. She continually scanned the area for her pursuers but saw no sign them. In truth, she wouldn't have recognized them if she had seen them. She'd been otherwise engaged during her escape and hadn't seen their faces.

The crowds on the waterfront were thinning, as was the traffic on Alaskan Way. The roaring sound of tires on pavement from the afternoon commute still filled the space over her head and around her with columns of vibrating air. The sun was low on the horizon, and the temperature was starting to drop. The winos in their huddled group a few pillars away no longer paid any attention to what she was doing.

Carrie knew she couldn't stay where she was much longer. She knew she was running out of options. She would have to move.

She slowly, very slowly, eased her way back up the cement support pillar; the adrenal hormones that she needed to maintain her blood pressure were still depleted, and it would take a moment or two for her sympathetic nervous system to take over. She felt light-headed.

The streetlights had blinked on, and soon it would be twilight. She took a deep breath and smelled the sea air. The light-headedness started to clear. She stepped out from the shadows toward Alaskan Way.

Carrie reached inside her pocket and removed her cell phone. The LCD indicated that it would need to be recharged soon. She reached back into her pocket and pulled out a piece of paper, and then she called the number she'd written there in the motel.

The dialed number started to ring as she walked out from under the viaduct onto the sidewalk. The Alaskan Way streetcar clanged as it rumbled by on its tracks. A foghorn sounded as the Bremerton ferry approached its dock. He answered her call after the fourth ring. Mavis had said that she could trust him. "This is Jon Kirk at the *Seattle Times*. I'm either away from my desk right now or on another line. Please leave a message after the beep, and I'll get back to you as soon as I can. If you need immediate assistance, press 0, and an operator will assist you.

"Beeeep."

"Damn!"

Carrie pulled the phone away from her ear. She needed immediate assistance; there was no doubt about that, but she wasn't about to press 0. Instead she broke the connection and put the phone back into her pocket. She thought for a moment and then started walking north along the waterfront toward the Edgewater Inn, an establishment dating from the time of the Seattle World's Fair.

She'd been walking for fifteen minutes or so when a cellular tower on top of the Space Needle transmitted a signal to the device in her pocket. Her phone started to ring. Her muscles involuntarily tensed, then relaxed as she realized that there must be a system tracking incoming calls at the *Seattle Times*. She retrieved the phone from her pocket, flipped it open, and pressed it to her ear.

"Hello?"

"Carrie Williams?" The voice was unfamiliar.

"Yes."

"Carrie, this is Chap Alvord. I'm a United States federal marshal."

There was a long silence.

"Carrie, are you there?"

Pause.

"Carrie, listen to me. It's very important that I talk to you."

More silence.

"Carrie, please, your life may be in danger. There are people from Florida ..."

Carrie stifled a scream. *Stupid, stupid, stupid!* She threw the still-open phone out into the oncoming traffic on Alaskan Way. It bounced off the front bumper of a dark-green pickup truck into the next lane of traffic, where it was smashed under the wheels of a Land Rover. The tires of subsequent vehicles then further crushed the smashed pieces.

A federal marshal? How could she be so dumb! They'd been monitoring her cell phone. If they could do it, potentially anybody could do it.

Carrie spun around. No one seemed to be watching her. She checked the other faces on the street. A bicycle messenger sped by. A pulsating bass from a muffled sound system thumped from a car stopped at a red light. Carrie picked up her pace. She walked as fast as she could without attracting attention to herself. A child asked her mother for an ice cream cone. Carrie turned right, away from the waterfront. She climbed up some steps toward Western Avenue and then up some more toward the Pike Place Market. She looked over her shoulder. No one had followed. She entered the market, working her way through its cloistered stalls. Smells of fish and fresh produce filled the air. She kept going.

# Chapter 20

KAREN ABLE HAD been working late. She was following up on her witness-protection-program angle and had run into more dead ends. Her contacts in the Justice Department had told her that Stewart Wolf hadn't been a protected witness. They assured her that even if someone had been protected under that pseudonym, there would be no reason to continue the charade now that he was dead. Still, what had she expected them to say?

She'd asked her departmental computer geeks to find out about the Total Information Awareness Program and had been told that a four-year time limit on information wasn't all that unusual—that it was a relatively new program and that data entry wasn't yet complete. They speculated that the system might have been prioritized for recent information first. Maybe Stewart Wolf wasn't a protected witness after all.

She was also tracing people who might have known about Candy Peterson's planned meeting with Jon, but she wasn't making much progress there, either. She was tired and twitchy, and she needed to burn off some energy. She took one last look at the notes in front of her, then put them away and left for the SPD gym in the basement. She'd just finished a workout with a jumping rope when she was summoned for a phone call.

There'd been a murder in Pioneer Square. A black male had been shot execution-style. He'd been bound, gagged, and taped to a rocking chair. He'd been shot twice, once in the head and once in the heart, with a small-caliber weapon. There were no exit wounds. "And get this," Robbie Washington said into his cell phone. "All of his fingers were broken."

Karen wiped the sweat from her face. "You've got to be kidding."

"Nope. Same M.O. as the Volunteer Park murder; probably the same perp or perps. The guy was tortured. Forensics and photographers are on the way. They should get here anytime now. You want to join the party?"

"Does a bear shit in the woods?"

"I thought so."

Karen reached for a towel. She patted her face, then her neck. "Tell me about the vic."

"His name was Chester Dorsey, an old guy, probably in his sixties. He was a musician. A neighbor found him here in his apartment. The front door was open when we got here. So was the back window; it leads to a fire escape. The neighbor says she was walking by and saw the open door. When she called out and no one answered, she stepped inside for a look. That's when she found him."

Karen continued to mop away her sweat.

"She looked around the apartment but says she didn't see anyone else there. She says she didn't touch anything. She isn't sure whether the back window was open when she was in there or not."

"Anything else?"

"Not really. She says she didn't see or hear anything unusual before she found the body. We're looking around for other possible witnesses, but so far nothing. We haven't found anyone willing to talk.

"Based on the state of his rigor mortis, Dorsey was killed several hours ago. The M.E. will give us a better time of death when she gets here."

Karen again patted her face with the towel. She was starting to cool down. "First Candy Peterson, then Chester Dorsey. Both were professional hits; both were tortured."

"Yup."

"What's the deal with the open door and window? That's not right. If the shooter was a pro, he would've taken care of business and then buttoned up the place. He wouldn't have left the front door open."

"We're working on that," Robbie answered. "Maybe forensics will give us an answer."

Karen thought about it for a moment. A strand of hair was sticking to the side of her face. She brushed it away. "Just exactly where are you?" she asked.

Robbie gave her the address.

"OK, stall the forensics people until I get there. I want first crack at the crime scene."

"They're not going to like that."

"Do what you've got to do. I'm on my way."

Karen hung up the phone. She jogged back through the acrid-smelling gym to the women's locker room, where she quickly showered and dressed. Then she rushed off for Chester Dorsey's apartment in Pioneer Square.

# Chapter 21

EVERY NEWSROOM HAS a pulse; you can feel it the moment you walk in the door. On slow news days the pulse is slow and steady. The accumulated sounds and muted conversations blend to form a kind of all-pervasive background white noise, a noise that seems to come from everywhere at once and nowhere in particular. It's a phenomenon somewhat analogous to the background microwave-radiation residual of the cosmic Big Bang, the backdrop against which the intensity of a news supernova can immediately be judged.

When Karen came home late the night before, after Jon had already gone to bed, the primordial ingredients for a cosmic event had already been mixed, and by the time Jon had left for work the next morning, before she got up, that pre-quark stew had started to boil. Twenty minutes later, when Jon arrived at the newsroom door, he was greeted by the Big Bang itself. Its pulse was fast, irregular, and explosive. Reporters were shouting, telephones were ringing, and chaos seemed to be expanding in a wavefront of action from Chris Collins, the city editor. Collins was at the epicenter. Jon saw him glare in his direction as he entered the room.

"Kirk, get in here! I want to talk to you." He strode off toward his office and nodded for Jon to follow. Then he slammed the door behind him.

Lizzy Carlstrom mouthed, "You're late." Jon acknowledged her comment with a half-smile. She shook her head and wagged her finger. Jon shrugged his shoulders.

Jean Viereck held up a copy of the morning *Seattle Post Intelligencer* with both hands. The headline spread across the front page in bold type read:

## MOB-STYLE MURDER IN PIONEER SQUARE
### By Jean Godden
*Seattle Post Intelligencer staff reporter*

"You've been scooped," she said. She too shook her head. Jon grabbed the paper out of her hands. He read the story as he neared Collins' office.

Vicki, Collins' secretary, tsk-tsked when he approached. "Watch yourself in there," she said. "He's really pissed."

"And I suppose this is all my fault?" Jon held up the paper. "It looks to me like everyone was scooped—the television networks, the wire services, talk radio, everyone. I'm not the only one."

"I wouldn't go in there with that attitude if I were you," she answered.

"What attitude?"

"That attitude."

Jon frowned, and then he opened the door to Collins' office.

:  :  :

Collins was sitting at his desk when Jon came in. He was

rereading the *P.I.* article. His lip was curled around an unlit cigarette. He didn't look up. Jon approached his desk and then stood there, waiting for Collins to say something.

"Do you remember the last time the *P.I.* beat us with an exclusive?" Collins finally growled. His nose was still in the paper.

"No," Jon answered, "I don't."

"Well, neither do I, Goddamn it!" Collins slammed the paper down. His eyes were fixed on Jon, and they were on fire.

"They beat us, Kirk, and they beat us bad. This isn't supposed to happen. We're the number-one paper in this town, not them! They're the out-of-town guys, the national chain that dallies in our market. Have you read this?" He pulled the cigarette out of his mouth and threw it in his wastebasket.

Jon said that he'd read part of it but that he hadn't had time to finish it all.

"Well, here," he shoved the paper across his desk, "read it."

"I've got my own," Jon said. He held up Viereck's copy of the *P.I.*

"Yeah? Well, hell of a way to get the news, isn't it!" Collins stood up and walked over to the water cooler in the corner. He filled a clear plastic cup with water, drank the whole cupful, threw the cup away, patted his shirt pocket for a pack of cigarettes, felt only Tootsie Pops, grunted something unintelligible, pulled one out, unwrapped it, and stuffed it in his mouth.

He was on his way over to the wastebasket to throw the wrapper away when Jon pulled one of the two chairs facing his desk to the side to sit down. Collins eyed him over the top of his Tootsie Pop stick. Jon looked into his eyes and decided it might be best to remain standing. Collins banked the wrapper into the wastebasket. "What are we going to do about this?" he asked. He moved back over to his desk. "We can't let this stand."

Jon responded with, "What do you mean?"

Collins' face turned red. "What do you mean, what do I mean? In case you haven't noticed, our circulation isn't what it used to be. The owners are going to bust my balls over this." He picked up the paper, looked at it, and suddenly pointed it at Jon. "Jean Godden's a great reporter," he said. "She's the best they have, maybe almost as good as you. She used to work for us before she went over to the dark side." He jabbed the paper at Jon like a rapier. "But she's not a Pulitzer Prize winner. Not like you. You're the one with the Pulitzer. You're the one who's supposed to be the hotshot around here. So tell me, how come she's the one who made the tie-in between Chester Dorsey and the Volunteer Park murder? How come her paper got the exclusive? I thought I could count on you for that sort of thing.

"Listen to this: *Both victims were killed in the same way with the same-caliber weapon. No shell casings were found at either crime scene. Both victims were tortured. Both had all of their fingers broken.*" Collins stopped for a moment and took a breath. He was staring at Jon. His lip started to twitch. His Tootsie Pop twitched with it. "This was supposed to have been your story," he said. "This should've been our exclusive, not theirs." He paused a moment. His lip twitched some more. "How am I going to make this place profitable with screw-ups like this? Where are my cigarettes?" He pulled open his top desk drawer, rooted around inside, and then slammed it shut.

Jon started to answer. "Uh ..."

Collins cut him off. "Jean Godden somehow got her story last night. Then she put it together and got it in to her editor by deadline. That's the way things are supposed to work. What were you doing last night? Where were you when all of this came down?"

"I, uh ..."

"Why didn't your girlfriend over at the SPD alert you about this? Was she too busy to call you, or what? Did you have a fight? You guys *are* sleeping together, aren't you?"

"Hey! Wait a minute! As I remember it, it was you who pulled me off the Candy Peterson murder story. I was too close to it. Remember? You gave me that stupid toilet-innovation piece instead. So don't look at me. You got a problem? Ask Lizzy! Maybe while you're at it, you ought to ask yourself! And as far as sleeping with my girlfriend ..."

"OK, OK, that was out of bounds, but I want to know what's going on! I want to know how Carrie Williams fits into all of this! I want to know who's behind these murders, and I want to know why! I want to know what really happened in Ocean City! And I want it printed in our paper before anybody else gets it, and that includes the electronic media and Jean fucking Godden! Get that?" He leaned forward across his desk. "Do you understand?"

"Yeah, I understand." They glared at each other for a few silent seconds. "But ..."

"But what?" Collins leaned a little farther forward.

The veins on Jon's neck popped out like a couple of blood-filled worms. He had an answer, but he squelched it; he knew he'd regret it. Instead he took a deep breath and replied, "Nothing!"

"Fine!" Collins leaned back in his chair. He pulled the Tootsie Pop out of his mouth. "Now get out of here." He stuffed the lollipop back in. "Bring me something tomorrow." His eyes dropped to his desktop. He pushed some papers around, looking for his pack of cigarettes.

"Tomorrow?"

"Yeah, tomorrow. We need a counter for that P.I. story." He grabbed the newspaper, buried his head in it, and again started to read.

Jon turned to leave the room and closed the door behind him. Vicki was still sitting at her desk working on her fingernails when he came out. "Didn't take my advice, did you?" She eyed him with an I-told-you-so look.

"You heard?" Jon asked.

"Of course I heard. I took the weather stripping out from around his door a long time ago. What kind of a secretary would I be if I didn't know what's going on around here?" She filed a nail for a few strokes and then added, "It sounds to me like you and your policeman girlfriend need to have a little talk. Isn't she supposed to be your source on the force?" She looked up innocently and then asked, "Are you guys still a thing, or is there something you'd like to tell me?"

"Vicki, look ..."

"Just looking out for your best interests, that's all," she said. She started to file her nails again. "I've got this friend, and, well, she's gorgeous. She's new in town, and I was thinking ..."

Jon shook his head as he walked back toward his desk. Vicki always had a friend. He sat down, turned on his computer, and checked his voice mail. There were twenty-three messages, too many for him to face all at once. He dispatched the first eleven and then called Karen. When he was informed that she was unavailable, he went back to get the twelfth. It was a hang-up. He checked his caller ID, and Carrie Williams' name popped into the LCD window. It also listed the number she'd called from.

Jon sat up straight. He immediately checked the time. The call had come in yesterday. He checked the origination number and pressed one to redial. The connection didn't go through. Instead a prerecorded message informed him that the cellular number he was calling wasn't available.

"Crap!" What was he going to do now? An interview with Carrie Williams would have gone a long way toward smoothing Chris Collins' feathers. He checked voice mail numbers thirteen and fourteen. Number fifteen was from Karen; she'd called earlier that morning to tell him about the *P.I.* story in case he hadn't already seen it. The department had wanted to keep it quiet until later today, and she had no idea who Jean Godden's contact was.

He dealt with the next five voice mails before getting another hang-up; the caller ID indicated a pay phone. It had come in less than an hour ago. There were two more hang-ups, each spaced about fifteen minutes apart, each from a pay phone. And then the telephone rang.

Jon reached for the receiver. His caller ID again indicated that the call originated from a pay phone. He pushed the flashing button on the incoming line. "Jon Kirk, *Seattle Times*." He heard a faint rustling noise, but no one spoke. He listened for a few seconds and then said, "Hello?" He waited for a few seconds more. He was just about to hang up when a voice answered:

"Hello? Jon Kirk?" The voice was not familiar.

"Yes, this is he."

"Jon, this is Carrie Williams. Mavis said you're one of the good guys. Are you?"

"Carrie ..." He fumbled for a note pad. He switched the receiver to his left hand and then picked up a pen in his right. He clicked down the point. "I try to be. Where are you?"

"I'd rather not say where I am right now, if you don't mind."

He got ready to write. "The whole world's looking for you, you know."

"I'm aware of that," she answered. "I'm in a bit of a bind. I was hoping you could help." He heard more of the rustling sound. It was a sound he knew but couldn't quite place. He was certain that he'd heard it before.

"Sure! Of course!" He wrote CARRIE WILLIAMS across the top of the pad and underlined it twice. "Anytime. What can I do for you?"

She paused a moment before she said, "Someone's trying to kill me."

"Someone's trying to kill …?" Jon's brain went into instant overload. Synapses fired. He wrote KILL on his note pad without consciously knowing that he'd done it. "Are you sure?"

"Am I sure? Well, let's see. Candy Peterson went to Seattle to tell you about Stewart Wolf and the bogus Dr. Bennett. Now she's dead. Chester Dorsey, an old friend, offered to help me and give me some advice. I came to see him. Now he's dead, too. And then there are the people who found me in Chester's apartment. They chased me down the fire escape and then all over the waterfront, and if they'd have caught me, I'd most certainly be dead like the rest of them. I just barely got away. Yeah, I think I'm sure."

Silence. Jon couldn't believe what he was hearing. Then he asked, "Do the police know about this?"

"About Chester's murder? Of course they do. It was in the morning paper, the other paper. About me being there shortly afterwards, I don't know. There were two of them, a man and a woman. The woman came into the apartment to get me. The man waited outside."

Jon started to write. After a second or two he asked, "Can you identify them?"

"You mean like in a police line-up? I don't think so. I saw them, but only while beating it out of there as fast as I could, and then only over my shoulder."

Jon's mind was racing. He had hundreds of questions. He had the exclusive he needed. "Carrie, would you mind if I recorded the rest of this conversation? I want to be sure I get it right and don't miss anything. No one else will hear it."

After a pause Carrie answered, "I'd prefer that you didn't."

"OK," Jon said, "no problem." He was speaking a little too fast. "I won't turn on the recorder. Only hand-written notes." He again heard the background rustling sound on the other end of the phone. It bothered him that he couldn't quite place it. He continued, "About your connection with Chester Dorsey ..."

"Maybe it would be better if we continued this conversation somewhere else," she said. "I'm not sure I'm comfortable talking about this over the phone. Maybe we should meet somewhere in person."

"Sure," Jon said. "Let's do that." He scribbled MEET on his note pad. "Let's meet in person. Where would you like to meet?"

"No tape recorders," Carrie said. "I don't want to have our conversation recorded."

"OK, no tape recorders. When could we meet? How soon? Where? If you'll tell me where you are, I can get there right away."

There was a few seconds' pause before Carrie answered, "I don't know." Then after another few seconds she said, "I'll let you know."

"Carrie?" Jon said.

The rustling sound abruptly stopped. She broke the connection. Jon blankly stared into the disconnected telephone receiver.

# Chapter 22

JON SMACKED THE receiver back down onto its cradle. His editor was on his ass, and he'd just screwed up a contact with Carrie Williams. He should never have mentioned the tape recorder. He leaned back against the back of his chair, puffed out his cheeks, and stared up at the ceiling for a few moments. Then he phoned the Seattle Police Department. Karen's direct line was busy, and he was immediately switched to her voice mail. She was talking to somebody else. Another frustration. He hung up the phone.

He decided to answer an earlier voice mail message. Chris Larson, the beer man from Safeco Field, had offered him a pair of Seattle Mariners tickets, box seats on the first base line. Chris was one of Jon's sports buddies. He sold hot dogs and beer at the baseball games and was able to wrangle free tickets from the team's ownership from time to time. Jon tried to call him back, but he couldn't reach him and had no way to leave a message. Chris was telecom challenged and computer illiterate. A third frustration. Jon decided to take a pass on the tickets.

He tried Karen again, and this time she answered the phone on the third ring. "Seattle Police Department. This is Detective Able."

"Karen, it's Jon."

"Jon, would you call me back? I can't talk right now. I'm in a meeting with Robbie. We're working on the Dorsey murder."

"Nice of you to let me in on that yesterday."

"Come on, Jon; you know how it works. We were supposed to keep it under wraps."

"Well, somebody didn't."

"Yeah, I know, but that somebody wasn't me. Now I really do have to go. Call me back later. I'll be free in an hour or so."

"Sure, I'll call you back later. And, oh, by the way, Carrie Williams was in Chester Dorsey's apartment yesterday. She just called. I suppose I should keep it under wraps, but since we're living together and all ..."

Silence.

"She says Dorsey was dead when she got there."

More silence.

"Someone surprised her while she was in his room and chased her down the fire escape. She thinks it must've been one of the murderers. She just barely got away."

Still more silence.

"It's a helluva story. The details will be in tomorrow's *Times*."

Deafening silence!

"Karen?"

"I'm here. Just give me a minute." A hand went over the receiver to muffle the sound; then a few seconds later, she said, "Where is she now?"

"I don't know. She wouldn't say. She wants to set up a meeting."

"When and where?"

"She wouldn't say. She said she'd let me know." Jon heard

Robbie's voice in the background.

"Did she tell you what she was doing in Dorsey's apartment, why she went there in the first place?"

"No, we didn't get that far. I didn't get a chance to ask."

"What about the people that were chasing her? Can she identify them?"

"She says no."

A hand again went over the phone. Jon heard a muffled discussion in the background. Then after several seconds Karen asked, "Do you know why she decided to call you and not the police?"

"I'm not sure."

Karen repeated his answer to Robbie. Jon heard "How convenient" and then more muffled conversation.

"Listen, Jon," Karen finally said. "If Carrie Williams calls you again, find out where she is, and then let us know right away. OK? Don't mess around with this on your own. She's part of a murder investigation; she's the common denominator between Candy Peterson and Chester Dorsey, not to mention Stewart Wolf and Linda what's-her-name. This is police business, not your business. Got that? I can't have you interfering with this investigation. You don't want to get caught obstructing justice. This is serious."

Pause.

"Jon?"

"Yeah, sure."

"Jon?"

"All right, I'll see what I can do, but it's a free country. She may not want to see you guys. You know how it is. That's her prerogative. There aren't any warrants out for her arrest, are there?"

"No, no warrants, and I understand that she still has her constitutional rights, but Jon, try to be a good citizen just this once, huh? OK? The cops are the good guys. We're all on the same side here."

"Uh … . OK, if you say so."

"Jon?"

"I said OK."

"Good. Now I really have to go. See you tonight?"

"I'll have a fire in the fireplace and a glass of wine waiting. We'll talk about it then."

"Great. I can't wait. I'll see you tonight. Bye."

"Bye." Jon hung up the phone. He had a faraway look in his eye.

:   :   :

Jon tried to work, but he couldn't concentrate. Carrie Williams' voice was like one of those songs you can't get out of your head. It kept circling around in his brain. He waited for her to call back.

He went through his e-mail and then scanned some online articles from the *L.A. Times* and *San Francisco Chronicle*. He glanced at his phone. He checked his watch. He looked outside through a window across the room. The sun was shining. The windowpanes were dirty. It looked like a nice day. He checked his watch again. Finally he gave up, stood, stretched, and turned off his computer. He was going home. He'd check for messages from Carrie from there.

He walked to his car. It was early, and traffic was light on Madison Avenue. He stopped at his favorite coffee shop for a double espresso and got into a heated discussion with the barista about a new Mariners starting pitcher; they needed a leftie, not another right-hander. He went back to his car and then turned toward his home on McGilvra Boulevard. He pulled into his garage, turned off the engine, and stepped out into his backyard. Then he stopped still. Adrenaline surged into his veins. He felt his breath catch. A six-foot-tall black woman was waiting for him on his deck.

"Carrie?"

Carrie had been sitting in a wooden lawn chair next to his hot tub. She stood when she saw him emerge from the back door of his garage. "That's right, Jon," she said. "It's me. I'm a little more put together than I was over the phone."

"Uh … . OK, how'd you get in here?"

"Sorry to startle you. It was just a little too exposed for me to wait for you out front. I hopped the fence."

"You didn't startle me." Jon had regained his composure. He walked across the yard onto the deck. "I'm glad you're safe."

"Yeah, me, too. I would've used the gate, but it was locked."

"Sorry about that," Jon answered. "I have a dog."

"I know. He keeps looking at me from out of the window. He probably wonders what I'm doing back here."

"Ah, I'd better let him out." Jon moved over to the back door. Leon came to the door as soon as he heard the key in the lock. He pressed his wet nose against the glass. When the door opened, he pushed his way through and immediately ran out into the yard to fertilize the garden. As soon as he'd finished, he came back to the deck to check out his new visitor. He began by sniffing her ankles, and then he sniffed up the side of her leg.

"Don't worry about him," Jon said. "He's very friendly. Just push him away if he bothers you."

"Oh, no bother. I love dogs." Leon looked at her with basset-hound eyes.

"Let's go inside." Jon opened the door for her and held it. She straightened up, brushed off her slacks, and followed him into the house. Leon stayed outside and cruised his yard.

Jon led her into his living room. "So how do we do this? He checked the street through his front window to make sure that it was clear and that she hadn't been followed. "Can I get you something before we get started?"

"No, thanks, I don't think so, not unless you happen to have an unassigned one-way ticket out of the country laying around here someplace. Rio's supposed to be nice this time of the year." She sat down on the couch.

"Sorry." He forced a smile. "A second choice?"

"Oh, maybe a Coke if you have one."

"I'll check." He went out into the kitchen, found two Cokes, and brought them back. He popped the tops and handed one to Carrie. "I should've asked if you'd like a glass, maybe some ice?"

"The can's fine," she said. "Thanks."

"OK then." He sat down on the other end of the couch, took a sip of his Coke, and put the can down on his coffee table. He turned toward her. There was an awkward few-second pause, then, "Where do we start? You're here to …?"

Carrie paused another moment. "You know, I'm not really sure. I hope I haven't made a mistake by coming here." She reached for her Coke. She felt better with something in her hand. "I want to find out about the things that have been happening to me. I want to clear my name, and Mavis told me you might help. I guess I should begin at the beginning."

Carrie started by describing her interactions with Bennett's impostor. "The cardiac-arrest code was a disaster. It shouldn't have happened." She told him about the subsequent hospital board inquest. "They suspended my hospital privileges and threatened my medical license. And then when my apartment was searched and Linda was murdered, I knew I had to get out of town. And finally, when Candy was tortured and killed ..." She told him how she hid out and made her way back to Seattle.

When Jon asked her about the Ocean City police, she demurred. "As far as I know, there isn't a warrant out for my arrest. They haven't contacted me."

"Maybe that's because they couldn't find you." Jon watched for a reaction. She didn't elaborate further. He assessed her body language. She appeared open and comfortable. She didn't fidget. She maintained eye contact, and her pupils were neither dilated nor constricted. Her blink reflex was normal, not excessive, and her skin appeared smooth and dry. He made a note. Then he asked, "Have you given any thought to why anyone would bother to use physician-assisted suicide as a tool for murder? Certainly there are easier ways to kill. In Linda's case they just snapped her neck. And as I understand it, Wolf would've lived only a few more weeks at most, anyway."

"I've thought about little else since it happened."

"It doesn't make any sense, does it? It's complicated and it's risky. It unnecessarily involves another person."

"Yes, that's true, but I have a theory." She moved toward Jon just a bit. "At first it didn't make any sense to me, either, but now, well, normally it'd be easy to murder someone in a hospital, especially someone who's been heavily sedated and restrained, someone who's essentially helpless. Our patient rooms are never locked, visitors are poorly monitored, and people can pretty much come and go as they please. There's no big-city-type security there, and as long as you're dressed appropriately and look like you know what you're doing, you can go pretty much anywhere you want. Nobody would notice a thing. In most cases it would be nearly impossible to know who's been in a patient's room during a particular segment of time."

Jon interrupted. "The digital tapes? The AV record-and-verify system?"

"That's right. You know about that?"

"Alex Morse mentioned it. Mavis knew about it, too. I'm a little confused about its purpose."

"Aren't we all? It was set up in a position to record his every movement and every word. It was supposed to be part of a new automated, comprehensive patient-monitoring system, but we all wondered about it.

"Wolf had a whole host of computerized physiological monitors and indwelling catheters set up to follow and record his medical status. He couldn't have hiccoughed without the computers knowing about it. There was no medical need for the AV stuff as far as I could see. It was an invasion of privacy. But it surely would've discouraged a potential killer from carrying out a murder, especially if he knew about the system ahead of time.

"I think that's what led to the physician-assisted suicide scheme. It's actually very clever when you think about it. Stewart Wolf obviously wasn't just an ordinary patient, not with the AV equipment and all. There had to be something else going on."

"I have my own suspicions about Mr. Wolf," Jon said. Although Karen had discounted it, the witness-protection program came to mind. "Let's fast-forward and talk about Chester Dorsey for a minute."

Leon trotted into the living room. He jumped up on the couch between Jon and Carrie, closer to Jon than to Carrie, and then he curled up and snuggled into the pillows.

"Chester Dorsey was a friend," she said, "a special friend. I'd known him all my life. He was my mother's lover and at times a surrogate father to me. I feel horribly responsible for his death." She told him about his offer to help her with her problems. She explained about how she'd climbed the fire escape to his apartment and about how she'd found him in his chair. "It was one of the worst moments in my life, second only to my mother's death." She was telling him about being discovered by one of his killers when Leon's tail began to wag. He jumped off the couch and ran out through the kitchen.

"Karen must be here," Jon said.

"Who's Karen?"

"Jon?" Karen said from the back door.

"In here," he answered.

Then from the back of the house, she yelled, "Cut it out, Leon! Jon, you've got to do something about this dog. He's humping again. Why can't you just take him over to that vet around the corner, what's her name, Shirley, and get him fixed? She's been after his nuts ever since she first laid eyes on him."

"Leon doesn't deserve that," Jon said. "He's a good dog."

"Well, if you're not going to get him fixed, at least take him to a doggie porno shop and buy him a blow-up leg or something. This is disgusting." She walked into the living room. Leon trotted in after her. "Oh," she said as she looked at Carrie with Jon on the couch. Jon stood when Karen entered the room.

"Carrie Williams, I presume?"

# Chapter 23

JON MADE THE introductions. "Carrie, this is Karen Able. She's a friend; she's also a Seattle police detective. Karen, this is Carrie Williams."

Karen's eyes were fixed on Carrie. She extended her hand. "Nice to finally meet you, Carrie," she said. They shook hands. "Jon's told me a lot about you. I'm the investigating officer on the Chester Dorsey and Candy Peterson murders. I've wanted to talk to you for some time now."

Carrie looked up at Jon. "Did you arrange this?" Her voice was cold.

"No, of course not."

"Then this is just a coincidence?"

"Look, Karen lives here, at least most of the time. She's not here as a cop. How could I have arranged this? I didn't even know you were going to be here."

Carrie said, "This isn't quite what I had in mind when I came." Then she turned to Karen. "Am I going to need a lawyer?"

"I don't know," Karen answered. Her eyes were still locked on Carrie's. "Are you going to need a lawyer?"

Carrie's change of expression was barely perceptible. Her

eyebrows arched a fraction of an inch, and her pupils constricted just a bit. She didn't answer.

"Hey," Jon said, "let's all relax here." His eyes shifted from Carrie to Karen and then back to Carrie. "Karen's not here to interrogate anyone. As I said, she's not here as a cop. And in any case, you won't need a lawyer. You're not a suspect in these crimes."

"Her fingerprints were found at the Dorsey crime scene," Karen said.

"Jesus, Karen, did you have to bring that up? I already explained that to you."

"You told her about our phone conversation?" Carrie asked. Her eyebrows went up a little farther. The cadence of her voice was slow. "I thought reporters weren't supposed to do that, to talk about their sources. I assumed that our conversation was confidential."

"Carrie, look, I'm trying to help. If you want me to treat something as off the record, just tell me, and I'll do it. I'll treat it as confidential. But you have to tell me what you want. I'm not clairvoyant."

"Jon," Karen interrupted.

"What?"

"Carrie and I need to talk. Why don't you and Leon go into the other room for a while? It won't take long, and it'll save us all a lot of trouble in the long run." She turned to Carrie. "OK?" She waited for an answer. When she got nothing back but an icy stare, she added, "We won't need any lawyers. This will be just between us." Still no answer. Carrie studied her for a moment before she finally nodded her head in agreement. Karen then turned to Jon. "OK, then, Jon, vamoose."

"Sure. It's getting a little testy in here, anyway." Jon left the living room for his study. "Come on, Leon."

Leon hopped off the couch, sat down for a moment to scratch behind his left ear, and then followed him out of the room.

:  :  :

"So now it's just the two of us," Karen said. "Tell me all you know about Stewart Wolf."

Carrie paused a moment and then asked, "From the beginning?" Karen nodded in the affirmative. Carrie sighed, "OK, from the beginning.

"Stewart Wolf. I wish I'd never heard that name." She started her story. "He was a man in the final stages of life. He had an incurable brain tumor, a glioblastoma multiforme. He knew he was going to die and that he didn't have much time left. He just wanted a little help with the process, that's all. That was his right under Oregon law."

"Is that what Dr. Bennett told you, or did Wolf tell you that himself?"

"Both. When Bennett, or whoever he really was, asked me to cosign the assisted-suicide papers, I told him I'd have to talk with my patient first. He agreed; he even encouraged it. Wolf was heavily sedated, so I gave him a stimulant to help bring him around. He never did fully wake up, but we communicated enough for me to understand that he knew he was going to die and that he wanted me to help him get it over with. His mind was slipping, he no longer had control over his bodily functions, and he was afraid of falling into a prolonged vegetative state.

"I don't know whether the living will he was supposed to have signed was real or not. It's since disappeared, but I'm absolutely certain that my actions were fully in accordance with his wishes and that he fully knew what he was asking me to do. There's no doubt in my mind that Stewart Wolf wanted me to help him die."

Karen eyed her for a moment. "As I understand it, the Sisters of Mercy held a board of inquest; they weren't so sure."

"They were just trying to cover themselves."

"I see. OK, we'll leave that for now." Karen flicked a strand of hair away from her face. "But then after the inquest, you left town and went into hiding. Why did you do that? The police had asked you to maintain contact, hadn't they?"

"You're kidding, right?"

Karen didn't answer. She just looked at her without changing expression.

"No, you're not kidding. Well, first there was Linda, and then Candy and Chester were killed. This is going to take a while."

And it did.

The interview took another hour to complete. When it was over, Carrie excused herself to go to the restroom, and Karen moved on into the study with Jon.

"Hi, babe," she said to his back. He was sitting at his desk, working on his computer.

Jon turned around. "How'd it go?"

"You never know," she answered. "But there is this. She says she was contacted by a federal marshal."

"A marshal as in a witness-protection-program marshal?"

"Could be. Anyway, she tells a good story. We'll check her facts, but my guess is that she's actually telling the truth. There are gaps, and not all of it makes perfect sense, but in general I think that things happened by and large the way she says they did. It's all too crazy for her to have made it up. If you can believe she was duped into the assisted-suicide scheme, then everything else flows from that. Now she's caught up in something that none of us quite understands, and she appears to be in real trouble. I hope she'll let us help her. I'm going to run it by Robbie tomorrow."

"I hope so, too," Jon said. He finished the sentence he was writing and then closed the lid to his laptop. "She seems like a nice person."

"Yeah, and not unattractive, either."

"I didn't notice."

"Uh-huh." Karen raised a well-practiced eyebrow. Leon looked at Karen's body language and perked up his ears. Jon scratched them back down.

"But you know what bothers me?" Jon continued. "How'd the people who killed Chester Dorsey know she was coming to Seattle? How'd they find out about the connection? They must've been waiting for her to show up. It's just a good thing that Chester told her to use the fire escape."

A voice came from behind him. "My cell phone." Jon swiveled his head. Karen turned around. Carrie stood at the doorway. Then she walked into the room and joined the group.

"Huh?"

"My cell phone," she repeated. "It had to be. There's no other way. I used a cell phone to call him from Portland."

"So you think somebody intercepted your cell call?"

"More likely they went through my phone records to get my contacts."

"It's easy to do," Karen added. "The information isn't supposed to be public, but anyone with a few connections and a little bit of guile could do it. And all they'd need is the information you get on your monthly phone bill. Which company do you use?"

"Verizon."

"OK, I'll do some checking tomorrow. Maybe I can find out who's been going through your records. In the meantime we'll need to find a place for you to stay, a place where you'll be safe."

"She can stay here," Jon volunteered. "She'll be safe here."

Karen's eyes flashed. "I'm not so sure that's such a great idea. Remember what we talked about? They've already made the connection between you and Carrie.

"Carrie, did you call Jon from your cell phone before you threw it away?"

Carrie glanced over at Jon. She winced as she answered, "Oh, God! I'm sorry."

Karen said, "Well, there's nothing we can do about that now." Then she continued, "You should be safe here, at least for tonight. I'm a light sleeper, and I'm armed, but tomorrow we're going to have to find someplace else for you to stay. Someplace a little less obvious."

Karen kept two nine-millimeter Berettas, and at least one of them was always close at hand and loaded. She also had handcuffs.

Loaded guns made Jon nervous. He never touched them, and he really wasn't sure what to think about having the Berettas in his house. He did, however, have some ideas about the handcuffs.

# Chapter 24

IT WAS 9:30 AM, and Jon was sitting in his back-bedroom office. He was working on his computer. Karen had left with Carrie at 7 AM. She'd taken her to SPD headquarters for a more formal interview, this time with Robbie, and then on to an undisclosed, supposedly safe location. Carrie's location would be revealed only on a need-to-know basis, and Jon was told that he didn't need to know. He wasn't to contact her without Karen's permission, and that wasn't likely. They'd argued and he'd lost. He was now officially out of the proverbial loop.

He finished what he was writing, scrolled down to the send icon, pressed the return key, and closed his laptop to put it to sleep. He'd just finished an article based on Carrie's interview and had sent it off to the newspaper. It would be his exclusive. Eat your heart out, Jean Fucking Godden! His editor would get a computer alert any moment now. He'd leave for work just as soon as he took Leon out for his morning walk.

Jon shaved, dressed, and picked up Leon's leash. Leon followed him out toward the front door. As they moved into the living room, Jon noticed a charcoal-gray Ford 500 slow and pull up to the curb in front of his house. He took a closer look out the window when it came to a complete stop. The driver-side front door opened, and a tall man in a dark navy suit got out. He seemed to check the address against a note he carried in his hand, and then he approached the house and rang the doorbell. Jon moved to the front door. He was in a hurry to get Leon's walk over with and to get to his office; he needed to talk with Chris Collins. He opened the door. "May I help you?" Leon peered out from behind his legs.

"Are you Jon Kirk?" He spoke with a mild Midwestern accent.

"I am." Jon's voice was curt; he was running late and was ready to brush him off. "Is there something I can do for you?"

"My name's Chap Alvord. I'm a United States federal marshal." Jon immediately flashed to thoughts of Carrie, her cell phone experience, Stewart Wolf, and the witness-protection program. Alvord reached into the left-hand breast pocket of his suit coat and removed his leather badge container. He flipped it open to show Jon his badge and ID. "May I come inside?"

Jon checked out the ID. It looked authentic enough. "Certainly."

"I'd like to talk to you about Carrie Williams, if you don't mind." He closed his badge container and replaced it in his pocket. "It shouldn't take too long." He took a half-step forward toward the door.

"Please come in."

Alvord stepped through the doorway. His suit was tailored and well pressed. He was wearing a white shirt with a light-blue patterned tie. His shoes were black, shined, Italian, and expensive, not thick-soled and dull like the ones the Seattle cops wore, and his strong, chiseled features and erect posture hinted at a military background. Leon sniffed the air as he walked by.

"You'll have to excuse me for a moment while I let my dog out in the backyard," Jon said. "He's long overdue. Why don't you have a seat and wait over there on the couch? I'll be back in just a minute or two." Jon motioned toward the couch. Then he led Leon through the dining room and kitchen and out through the back door into the yard. When he returned, Alvord was still standing, looking at a primitive tribal mask hanging on the wall.

"It's from Brazil," Jon said to his back. "It's a souvenir; it came from the Holyoke Collection."

Alvord turned around. "You have a very nice place here. How long have you owned it?"

"Three years," Jon answered. "It's been a good investment." He moved farther into the living room. "But then you're not here to talk about real estate, are you?" He led him toward the couch. "Should we start with Carrie Williams, or instead maybe the witness-protection program? Stewart Wolf was in the witness-protection program, wasn't he?" He watched for a reaction. Alvord gave him almost none. "That's what federal marshals do, isn't it? Protect witnesses?"

Alvord sat down on the couch. Jon sat at right angles to him in a chair. After a pause Alvord finally said, "You know I can't answer that. Why would you even ask?" His eyes were unblinking. They were firmly fixed on Jon's.

"Well, let's see," Jon answered. "You're a U.S. marshal. Wolf, a hotshot hospital consultant totally unsuited to the community, moves to a small out-of-the-way coastal town in Oregon. He doesn't seem to have much of a personal history. His records in the Total Information Awareness Program go back only four years. He was murdered under unusual circumstances, with Carrie

Williams the instrument of his demise. You want to talk to me about Carrie and presumably the murder. I'm a reporter. What am I supposed to make of all this? It's my job to ask questions."

Alvord's lip twitched. He sat back in his seat and put his elbow on the armrest. "Well, well, well, isn't this interesting?" He looked away for a few seconds while he pondered what to say next, and then he shifted his gaze back to Jon. He chose his words carefully.

"OK, Jon, you're a smart guy. Tell me, if I were to confirm your suspicions, on background and off the record, of course, what would you be willing to do for me in exchange?"

Jon felt an adrenaline rush. "That depends."

"It depends?" He stared at him for a few moments. "I hardly think so, not with your reputation." He paused a second or two, waiting for an answer. Hearing none, he continued, "Well, then, since dead men tell no tales, at least not on the witness stand, I guess there's no harm in telling you that Stewart Wolf *was* a protected witness. That deception no longer seems to be necessary, does it? Stewart Wolf, of course, wasn't his real name."

Jon nodded. "Of course not. His real name was ...?"

"We'll talk about that in a minute." Alvord shifted a little to the side. "But first I have a question for you. How did you gain access to the Total Information Awareness Program? The system is protected; it wasn't exactly designed for reporters, you know."

"Karen Able, she's a detective with the SPD. She has authorized access. She was working with it and told me about the information block at four years."

"Detective Able." He nodded. "I see." His eyes defocused for a moment, as if he were thinking about something else. "We'll have to work on that." He thought a moment more. "Still, that couldn't be how Wolf's cover was blown, could it?"

"Wolf's cover was blown?" Jon's voice trailed off.

"We're talking about the person or persons responsible for Stewart Wolf's murder, the people who duped Carrie Williams into killing him. She was just a pawn in all of this, you know. She's only a minor player."

"I doubt if she sees it that way," Jon said as he sat back in his chair. After a few seconds of silence he continued, "I assume, then, that you agree with Carrie Williams' version of events."

"Oh, absolutely," Alvord answered. "We have no doubts about it."

"Then she's not in any trouble, not with you or any other legal authority?"

"I wouldn't say she isn't in trouble," he answered. "She may not be in trouble with the law, but she certainly has her problems. We have reasons to believe that Stewart Wolf's murder was arranged by members of a Miami crime syndicate. We believe that Carrie Williams' life is in real danger. We'd like to talk with her about that, among other things. It's very important that I find her. I assume that you know where she is."

Jon shook his head. "Unfortunately, no, I don't," and he didn't. "She did contact me, though," he added. "She told me that someone was after her and that she thought her life was in danger. She wanted me to write her story." He wasn't yet ready to tell Alvord that he could contact her through Karen.

"And you wrote it?"

"I wrote it as she told it. I verified as much as I could. It's already filed. You can read it in tomorrow's paper."

"Would you show it to me? I assume you can get me a preprint."

"No problem. I'll print one up from my computer. It may not be exact—my editor has to review it—but it'll be close. Do you want me to do it for you now?"

"Not right now," Alvord said. "I'll get it later. You based it on a telephone interview?"

"No, I did the interview in person."

The corner of Alvord's lip again twitched. "In person?"

"Yes, in person. Carrie surprised me here at my house yesterday afternoon. She was waiting for me here when I came home from work. I had no idea ahead of time that she was going to be here. She was waiting in the backyard."

Alvord studied his face as he asked, "And you're sure you don't know how to contact her?"

"No, I'm sorry, I really have no idea where she is. She said she lost her cell phone."

Jon heard some scratching in the background. "Excuse me a moment." He stood up. "Leon's at the back door. I'd better let him back inside. I'll be right back." He walked out into the kitchen, stood by the door for a few seconds puzzling over something, and then let Leon in. "Can I get you anything while I'm out here?" he asked from the kitchen. "Some coffee or some juice, maybe some water?"

"No, no, thank you."

"Suit yourself." Jon filled a glass with tap water, quickly drank it, and returned to the living room. He sat down, looked at Alvord, and without wasting any time asked, "So are you going to tell me now who Stewart Wolf really was?"

"You have no idea?"

"No," he said. "Not yet, but while I'm on a roll … . In addition to his real identity, where did he come from?  Why did he need your protection? Who were you protecting him from, and how did Carrie get involved?"

He chuckled. "You don't really expect me to answer all of that, do you?"

"Why not? What could it hurt?" He cocked his head slightly to the side. "Wolf's dead. It's all going to come out anyway. Someone's eventually going to report the story. Why not me?"

A hint of a smile crossed Alvord's face. "Yes, indeed, why not you? But as I said, I need something in exchange. There's a price to be paid."

"A deal?" Jon asked.

Alvord glanced out through Jon's front window. A young mother was walking her baby in a stroller across the street. "Yes, a deal." He focused back on Jon. "I need you to connect me with Carrie Williams."

Jon answered without hesitation, "I can do that. No problem. Listen, you tell me about Stewart Wolf, and I'll connect you with Carrie Williams just as soon as she calls. She's bound to contact me after she sees the article in tomorrow's paper. I'll have her call you right away."

Alvord folded his hands into a prayer-like position, brought them up to his lips, and rested his chin on his thumbs while he turned his attention away from Jon and again out the front window. The woman with the stroller was gone. Jon waited for a response. Finally Alvord looked back at Jon over his folded hands. "Remember, this is on background."

"Of course."

"You can quote a highly reliable source in the Department of Justice."

"Whatever you say."

"And you'll do more than just ask Dr. Williams to call me when she contacts you. You'll set up a meeting, and you'll see to it that she shows up, too."

"I'll do my best."

"You'll set up a meeting at a place of my choosing, and you'll see to it that she shows up in person. I want to meet with her face to face."

"I'll take care of it."

"You'll do more than your best to take care of it. You'll see to it that she's there. That's an absolute requirement."

"Consider it done. I'll set it up. She'll be there. Don't worry."

"Her life may depend on it."

"I believe you. Based on what she's told me, I believe you."

"OK, then," he said, "here's your story. Alvord sat back in his chair and took a deep breath. Then he began.

"Stewart Wolf's real name was Frankie Wolfson; he was a numbers guy, an accountant, and he worked for the Grinstein crime syndicate in Miami. If you haven't read about him, you should have."

"The name sounds familiar. Everyone knows about the Grinstein crime syndicate."

"OK. Well, anyway, Frankie was busted about a year and a half ago in a Medicare sting operation. It was a really big deal at the time; it still is. It was the first case of its kind, the first one linking a big-time crime syndicate to a big-time organized health care fraud.

"Medicare fraud is a multibillion-dollar-a-year industry in this country. Organized crime couldn't pass up an opportunity like that, and Frankie, as it turned out, was right in the middle of it all. The government had set up a task force to work the problem, and in the end they were more than willing to trade Frankie his freedom for information about, and testimony against, his organization.

"Frankie was the Grinsteins' bookkeeper, and although he wasn't officially a 'made man' in the old Mafia sense of the term, he did know everything there was to know about their Medicare operation. He knew who was involved, who did what to whom, and how they did it. And most importantly, he knew where the money was. In the end, it didn't take much to get him to turn on his friends. Frankie wasn't all that enamored with the thought of hard time in a federal prison. I'll tell you more about that in a minute."

"Now I remember," Jon interrupted. "It was in the national news for at least a week. His friends in the syndicate swore he'd never live to testify."

"That's right, but the story really starts way before that. It started several years ago when a man walked into a Citibank branch in Miami and asked to withdraw $78,000 from his bank account. He'd opened the account two-and-a-half weeks earlier under the name of C. Calvert Knudson and had deposited somewhere in the neighborhood of $600,000 in Medicare checks during the first ten days that it was open. They were all made out to a New Jersey radiologist as reimbursement for various services rendered.

"During one of his visits to the bank, a teller noticed that the man in front of her resembled a John Doe she'd recently seen on a Citibank security flyer. The office of the inspector general at Health and Human Services had suspected him of perpetrating a series of Medicare frauds, and they'd been looking for him for more than a year. He'd apparently used several aliases, and his real name was unknown.

"A month earlier the same John Doe had walked away from over $300,000 in a Charles Schwab account when the Social Security number he provided turned out to be false. The manager from the brokerage house had phoned him to ask him a few questions, such as Did he have a medical license number? Did he have a Bureau of Narcotics and Dangerous Drugs number? Did he know what the acronym AMA stood for?

"John Doe didn't waste any time. He quickly hung up the phone and vanished. He left his money behind.

"Following the incident at Schwab, John Doe stepped up the pace of his operations. He began to withdraw millions of dollars deposited in various bank and brokerage accounts under various names all over South Florida. HSS agents, police officers, and bank officials started tracking him, but they were always just a step or two too slow. He was finally caught when that astute teller at Citibank signaled a security officer, who in turn notified the FBI, who got a police officer to the bank in time to cuff the subject and make an arrest. John Doe was still waiting at the teller window for his cash when the cops arrived.

"John Doe turned out to be Ron Barclay, a two-bit hood loyal to the Grinstein crime syndicate. He was sentenced in October to two-and-a-half years in a federal penitentiary. He never said a word during his trial, even though it would've knocked time off his sentence, and it was only by luck that we eventually connected him with Frankie Wolfson. With the exception of the $78,000 from Citibank, none of the millions he withdrew from any of the area financial institutions has ever been found."

"Excuse me a minute," Jon said. "I need to catch up. You're talking too fast." He'd been taking notes on the note pad he'd taken from the corner table. He scribbled something else and then flipped the page. "There, that's it. Go ahead."

"OK, the General Accounting Office reports that health care fraud consumes at least ten percent of the $1 trillion Americans spend on health care every year; that's $100 billion a year, and even that figure is probably too low. Other reports peg health care fraud as high as fourteen percent, or $140 billion. It's no wonder that organized crime is involved with this business. The narcotics business, by comparison, is significantly more dangerous and has estimated annual U.S. sales of only $65 billion. There are those who say that if we could only solve the health care fraud problem, we could pay off the national debt.

"The kinds of Medicare fraud most commonly perpetrated by organized crime are all based on identity theft. All they really need is a patient's Social Security number, a doctor's Medicare-provider number, a computer to generate bogus bills, and a post office box to receive the checks. The Barclay connections alone involved over thirty bogus companies, companies like surgical supply houses, orthopedic shoe companies, radiology clinics—you name it. By the time he was finally caught, he'd billed the government for several hundred million dollars. And Barclay was just a foot soldier. So far we've been able to trace over five hundred phony clinics and incorporated suitcase companies to the Grinstein crime syndicate. We're sure there are more. If you want to go out and steal, say, half a billion dollars, there's probably no easier or safer way to do it than through fraudulent Medicare bills."

Jon held up his hand and interrupted him. "How do these guys get their hands on all those doctor Medicare-provider numbers and patient Social Security numbers? It can't be all that easy, at least not in the numbers that we're talking about here."

"They have informants inside insurance companies. They have connections in virtually every aspect of the health care industry. Remember, we're talking about organized crime here, and it's very well organized indeed. Many South Florida drug traffickers have given up their drug business and diversified into health care fraud. They find it a lot safer and more lucrative than their usual line of work, and they bring their drug-business tactics of physical violence and intimidation with them.

"But back to the story. Following up on complaints from patients whose insurance companies had been billed for services that they'd never received in states that they'd never even been to, investigators found that the reimbursement checks had been sent to thousands of $10-per-month private rented mailboxes all over South Florida. Trying to stake out all of those mailboxes would've been a nightmare, so instead of the mailboxes, we began to track the checks themselves."

"Which *we* are we talking about here?" Jon asked.

"The Justice Department. That includes the FBI. It was with the help of the Florida State Banking Commission, however, that we got our first real break. Through surveillance cameras monitoring teller cages, we were able to collect the identifications John Doe had used to open up his multiple bank and brokerage accounts. And then at least his face, if not his name, had come into focus. The teller recognized him because bank security had sent the flyers around."

"And then you got him, but what does Barkley have to do with Wolf, or Wolfson?"

"We connected them through his girlfriend. Her name was Barbara Svoboda, and like a lot of those gangster molls, she was a little short of brains. On the other hand, she was a Playboy bunny type and had a body that wouldn't quit. When we contacted her about her boyfriend, all she did was bawl her eyes out. He was in jail, and she was too upset to talk. She was totally full of shit, of course. Her house was a mess. But when we returned a day later with a search warrant, the house had been cleaned out. All that was left was a desk and a few pieces of furniture. It had been sanitized—almost, anyway. Incredibly, there was an ink blotter left on the desk with a name and telephone number scribbled on the back. Svoboda must've left it there on purpose; maybe she had a grudge or something. We'll never know for sure. Who knows what really goes on inside those mobster families? Anyway, the name on the back was Frankie Wolfson, and the number was his cellular telephone number. That was the connection we needed. Needless to say, we gave him a call."

"Hold on a second," Jon said. He scribbled for another thirty seconds or so, and then he said, "OK, go ahead."

"OK, Frankie lived in Naples, and he lived very well indeed. He had an eight- thousand-square-foot house on an Oceanside estate with outbuildings and an Olympic-sized swimming pool. He was thought to have made his money as a high-profile hospital consultant.

"When we checked him out, he was indeed a financial consultant to many of the larger hospitals around the state, and his income taxes accurately reflected his detectable income and his lifestyle. When we asked him about Ron Barclay, he stated that he'd never heard of him and that he had absolutely no idea how his name and telephone number came to be written on the back of an ink blotter in his house. Surveillance did reveal the occasional contact with known members of the Grinstein crime syndicate. These contacts, however, were almost always limited to some sort of social situation or other, usually at one of his clubs. Business was never discussed at these meetings.

"Anyway, after several of these recorded contacts, and after an effort to find just the right judge, we were able to obtain a search warrant to search his property. It took us two days, but on the afternoon of the second day, bingo! We struck the mother lode. A magnetometer discovered a strong contact beneath the oak flooring of his extensive wine cellar. We pulled back a carpet and removed some loose planking to discover a substantially sized hidden safe. The safe was opened and documents were removed. Not only did we discover that he was the Grinstein syndicate's chief accountant, but we also discovered that he'd been skimming a not-insignificant portion of their profits into his own accounts, and by not insignificant I mean in excess of one hundred million dollars. We knew right then that we had him and that he would turn. There was no way he could've survived in federal prison after having ripped off the Grinstein syndicate.

"Frankie had a collection of templates for phony physician prescriptions and physician certificates of medical necessity for equipment—equipment like wheelchairs and prostheses that were paid for by Medicare but never delivered to unsuspecting patients. He'd designed a scam to give elderly patients air conditioners, TVs, blankets, pillows, and even angora-wool long underwear in exchange for their Medicare numbers and an agreement to visit certain doctors who then fabricated diagnoses and reported faked accidents. He'd invented more than five hundred bogus laboratories and had records of tens of thousands of stolen patient identities. He'd worked out a program to provide free physical examinations to health club members, requesting their insurance information as background and then stealing their health care billing information. Literally billions of dollars were billed through these schemes; we still aren't sure exactly how much. And only Frankie knew how much was actually collected and laundered. It was the biggest health care rip-off in the history of health care rip-offs."

Jon looked up from his note pad. "So where's the money now?"

"Who knows? It's gone. Frankie laundered it, but in the end he turned it over to someone else, a good business practice on the part of the Grinstein syndicate. He said that he laundered it through the Bahamas after Castro shut down his Cuba connections, but that he had no idea where it went after that. We've tried to trace it, but so far all we've been able to recover is a little over two million dollars. That's not chump change, mind you, and it's enough to put several members of the Florida syndicate in jail for a very long time, but it's nothing when compared to the billions of dollars that were stolen.

"And as for Frankie's money, he says that's gone, too. According to his lawyer, all he had at the time we arrested him was about $14,000 in his checking account and several million in stocks and bonds, all attributable to his hospital consulting business. We'd planned to let that part of it slide until he'd completed his testimony against the Grinstein syndicate."

"But now he's dead."

"Yes, now he's dead."

"And now you have neither the testimony nor the money."

"Thanks for pointing that out."

"And I suppose this brings us up to the point where Carrie Williams became involved."

"Not quite. You see, the price for securing Frankie's

commitment to testify against his friends was a new identity and no jail time. The AG approved the deal. Even his lawyer didn't know about it, since he too was connected to the Grinstein syndicate. Anyway, we got Frankie into the program and got him a job. He was hired as a consultant to the Sisters of Mercy Medical Center. This arrangement offered him a legitimate source for a substantial income and also an opportunity to channel his considerable energy into his chosen field of expertise. There are scads of hospital consultants around the country, and the whole thing was to be kept low profile.

"It all worked well for a while, too. Frankie made his consulting money, and his cover identity seemed secure, but as his situation evolved, it turned out he was a little too good at his job. With Frankie's advice, Alex Morse was able to save her failing hospital, and she became the darling of the hospital administrator world. He taught her how to turn a loser hospital into a total money machine. It brought undue attention to the little town of Ocean City. And then he got cancer, and then someone from his old crime syndicate must've discovered his identity, and that's what brings us up to the point where Carrie Williams became involved."

Jon sat back in his chair. He cracked his back. He put down his pen and flexed his fingers. Alvord glanced at his watch. "Uh-oh, it's later than I thought. I have an appointment downtown in the federal building in forty-five minutes, and I don't want to be late."

Jon picked up his pen and note pad and said, "OK, let's wrap it up."

"OK, then, as I was saying, Frankie got cancer, brain cancer, and it was incurable. He was going to die, and he knew it. We tried to move up the date of the trial, but the other side just wouldn't play ball, and in the process of dealing with the court, we may've inadvertently tipped off his friends to his medical condition. With that information, and with the Sisters of Mercy Medical Center's newfound notoriety as a profit center, it was only going to be a matter of time before they'd find him. But when they finally did, it was already too late. He was in the hospital and only semi-lucid. He was on painkillers, among other things, and there was no way they could interrogate him. So all there was left to do was to take care of business and finish him off before he could say anything about their money.

"Meanwhile, Alex Morse had set up that extensive audiovisual system in his hospital room. Her reasons for installing it are still unclear; maybe she suspected something. I'm not sure. We've asked her about it, and she's been vague, but whatever the reason, that system would've made it difficult for a hit man to do his job and get away with it. A professional would've cased the place ahead of time and would've had to have found out about it." Alvord stopped for a minute, waiting for Jon to catch up and stop writing. When he saw that Jon had finished, he said, "And then, as for Carrie Williams, well, I believe she's told you the rest.

"Now I've got to get out of here or I'll be late."

"Whew," Jon said. "What a story."

"Yes, isn't it?" He reached into his right-hand breast coat pocket and pulled out a card. "Here's my card." He handed it to Jon. "Call the number listed there any time of the day or night. I want to know it the minute you hear from Dr. Williams. I want you to arrange a meeting, and then I want you to call me. I'll set up the time and place. You'll call her back with the details, and you'll make sure she shows up. Do you understand?"

Jon answered, "I understand."

Alvord locked onto Jon's eyes with his own. "This is our deal, and I expect you to honor it."

"Don't worry," Jon said. "I will. You just gave me the story of the year."

# Chapter 25

JON SHUT THE DOOR, hurried back across the living room, and picked up his notes. Stewart Wolf was Frankie Wolfson. He really was a protected witness. Carrie was innocent. And the Grinstein syndicate was in Seattle. He had to call Karen. He reached for the telephone and dialed her work number.

A recorded voice answered, "Seattle Police Department, Detective Lieutenant Karen Able. I'm away from my desk right now. Leave a short message after the beep and I'll get back to you. If this is an emergency, or if you'd like to talk with another officer, please … ."

Jon hung up the receiver. He tried her cellular number but got no answer there, either. It had been turned off. "Sorry, Leon," he said as he stood up. "No time for a walk today. Maybe this evening." He bent over and scratched him on the head. Then he walked to the kitchen, picked up his keys, and left the house. He called Chris Collins on his way to work. Vicki answered the phone.

"*Seattle Times*, Mr. Collins' office, Vicki speaking. May I help you?"

"Vicki, it's Jon." He told her to hold the Carrie Williams story.

"What?"

"Tell Collins to hold it, not to print it. I've got something else; it's better. We'll run it instead of the other one. And, Vicki, tell him he might have to be a little flexible with the deadline."

"Are you kidding me? That costs money. He'll never do that."

"Tell him I'll be there in twenty minutes. I'll explain when I get there."

"OK," she said. "I'll tell him, but this had better be good."

Jon knew that it was a lot better than good.

:     :     :

Jon drove up Madison Avenue and then cut across Capitol Hill to Denny Way. He followed it all the way down to the *Seattle Times* building. He was speeding, weaving through the mid-day traffic, and it still took him twenty minutes to get there. After parking his car and traversing security, he jogged up the stairs to the newsroom. As he approached Vicki's desk, she pursed her lips and said, "Go on in; he's expecting you." Jon opened the door.

"Kirk!" Collins was sitting behind his messy desk. He'd been popping jellybeans into his mouth. "Where've you been? What's going on?" Why shouldn't we print your story? It's damn good! And what's this about the deadline?"

"Mind if I sit down?" Jon asked.

"No, go ahead. Want a jellybean?" He held out a bowl of jellybeans in Jon's direction.

Jon pulled one of the chairs facing Collins' desk to the side and sat. "No, thanks." Then he told him about the U.S. marshal's visit to his house.

He told him that Stewart Wolf was really Frankie Wolfson and about the witness-protection program. He described the way the Florida syndicate ran its Medicare fraud operations, and the way billions of dollars had been laundered and was still missing. He told him about the audiovisual equipment in Frankie's hospital room and then about Carrie Williams' part in it.

"You're shitting me!" Collins said.

"I shit you not. This is the story of the year." Jon told him about the money that Frankie had skimmed from the Grinstein syndicate and about how all of that was also still missing.

"How the hell did you get all this? U.S. marshals just don't do this sort of thing for no reason."

"We made a deal," Jon said. "Alvord wants a meeting with Carrie Williams. He wants me to set it up."

"And you can do that?" He pushed the jellybeans away, reached into his desk, and pulled out a package of cigarettes.

"I can."

"You're sure? It all sounds too easy, too pat." He pulled a cigarette out of the pack. "You're sure this guy's really who he claims to be?" He put it between his lips.

"His ID looks good. I think he's real, but of course I'll check him out. I'll call the Justice Department just as soon as we're finished here." Jon straightened the chair. "But assuming he checks, what about the deadline?"

Collins felt his pockets for a match and, finding none, pulled the cigarette out of his mouth by its tip, looked at it, and then put it down on his desk. "You don't happen to have a match, do you?" Jon just looked at him. "No, of course you don't." He again looked at his cigarette. "Look, you write the story, and I'll make a few phone calls. I'm not promising anything, but I'll see what I can do."

"Thanks, boss." Jon almost never called him boss. "You won't regret it."

"I hope not."

Jon thanked him again. Then he hurried out of the office and pulled the door closed behind him.

:     :     :

Jon walked over to his desk, turned on his computer, and grabbed a triangular piece of wood out of a drawer. It was mounted with a brass plaque that read, "DON'T TALK TO ME." He put it on top of his computer monitor. The all-pervasive din of the newsroom seemingly melted away into nothingness.

He called the local offices of the Justice Department and asked if they had a U.S. Marshal Chap Alvord working there. He was put on hold for a few minutes and then was told that a Marshal Alvord was assigned to the Portland office. He asked them if they had a photo, then described Alvord: taut features, strong jaw, salt-and-pepper hair, handsome. They confirmed that his description matched their photo. His unnamed Justice Department official checked out.

Next he wrote Carrie Williams, Frankie Wolfson, Witness Protection Program, Medicare Fraud, Florida Crime Syndicate, Candy Peterson, and Chester Dorsey each on a separate yellow Post-It Note and stuck them all on the surface of his empty desk. They were the pieces of his puzzle, and he moved them around to visualize how they fit. There was Alex Morse and the hospital's integrated audiovisual patient-monitoring system. He started making connections. Finally he started to type. And although he didn't finish until well after deadline, Collins assured him that his article would appear in the next day's paper. Then he leaned back in his chair, arched his back, stretched, and did what he always did after he finished a big story. He left the office and drove across town to a sleazy little place in one of Jairus Stratton's run-down buildings just a mile away from the university, the Blue Moon Café.

# Chapter 26

THE BLUE MOON CAFÉ really wasn't much of a café; in fact it wasn't a café at all. It was a dingy, semi-notorious, slightly over-the-hill bar that catered to a loyal crowd of regular customers and an occasional university student, and it was one of Jon's favorite places in the world. The café part of the title was added in a not-so-subtle attempt to get around some of Seattle's more-antiquated blue laws. Jon had discovered the place years ago while in journalism school at the University of Washington. Bobby Arnold, its long-time bartender and a permanent fixture around the place, greeted him as he walked in the door.

"Jon, where've you been? We haven't seen you around here for at least a couple of weeks." His practiced hand reached behind the bar, grabbed a glass, and filled it with Redhook from the tap.

"I've been kind of busy." Jon picked up the beer as Bobby slid it to him. "The Peterson and Dorsey murders have been keeping me out of trouble."

"Yeah? I've been reading about that. You've written some good stuff."

"You ain't seen nothin yet!" Jon slugged down a gulp of beer.

Redhook was Jon's favorite beer, and Bobby Arnold was Jon's favorite bartender. A sign behind the bar read:

## IF YOU THINK NOBODY CARES, TRY SKIPPING A PAYMENT.

Jon took another sip of his beer. Bobby pulled a towel out from behind the bar and started wiping a watermark from its polished surface. He'd been following Jon's series of articles. "How are you coming with that nasty bit of business down in Ocean City?" he asked. "You still think Carrie Williams is mixed up with the Peterson and Dorsey murders? Your articles were a little less than conclusive." When Jon told him about Alvord's visit, he said, "Ooowee! A doc conned into killing her own patient, who just happens to be a protected witness in an organized crime case. You don't see that every day."

"No, you don't," Jon answered. "Read about it in tomorrow's paper. Spend a quarter and buy a copy."

"I have a subscription."

"So do I." It was Carla Frehse, a regular Blue Moon customer sitting at the far end of the bar. She was by herself, drinking a Manhattan.

"You're one of the few who still do," Jon said in response. He lifted his glass in a mock toast. She toasted back. Bobby kept working on the watermark.

Carla put her drink down and slowly began stirring it with her index finger. "You know your doctor's guilty as hell, don't you?" She pulled her finger out of her drink and sucked off the alcohol. "She murdered that guy in the hospital, pure and simple. Anyone with half a brain can see that." She put her finger back in her Manhattan and started stirring again. "She gets away with it,

210 THOMAS W. GRIFFIN

too; the pretty ones always do. I saw her picture." She looked at Jon in a seductive sort of way. "You guys are all the same when it comes to nubile bodies."

Jon turned to face her. "Nubile?"

Bobby ignored her. "What does SPD think? Karen's supposed to be working on the case, isn't she? What does she think about your new information?"

"Karen? Oh, shit! I forgot to call her back. She's the lead detective, and she doesn't know. She's going to kill me." Jon stood up, pulled his cell phone out of his pocket, and speed-dialed Karen's number.

:   :   :

Karen was in her office when she got the call. Robbie was with her. They were discussing their interview with Carrie when her cell phone chimed. "Hi, Jon." She pressed her hand over the talk end of the phone and whispered to Robbie, "It's Jon. I'll just be a second. Don't leave." Then she took her hand away and said, "Listen, I'm kind of busy right now. Could you ..."

Jon told her about his conversation with Marshal Alvord. "What?" He told her about his call to the Justice Department. "Your description matched their photograph?" He told her that Stewart Wolf was really Frankie Wolfson. "So he *was* in the witness-protection program." He told her that Carrie wasn't wanted anywhere for anything. "I already know that." He mentioned the Grinstein syndicate. "The Grinstein syndicate? They're a fusion organization, the future of organized crime. Members come from the old Italian Mafia, the Russian mob, Cubans, Colombians; you name it. They're all involved. Jerry Grinstein is the FBI's unstated public enemy number one; they just haven't been able to pin him with anything yet. They'd sell their souls to put him behind bars. It's only a matter of time before we see that sort of thing here in Seattle." Then he told her about his deal with Alvord.

"You shouldn't have promised him that. Your direct contacts with Carrie Williams are over; they go through me now. Her whereabouts are no longer your concern. He should've called us, not you."

"He probably got my name from a cell phone trace."

"Why didn't you tell him we're protecting her?"

"I don't know. I just didn't."

"Well, I hope it wasn't just because you wanted to stay involved, because that's not going to work."

Robbie said something in the background; then Karen asked, "Where are you now?"

Jon answered, "I'm with Bobby at the Blue Moon."

"The Blue Moon? Good. My favorite sleaze bucket. Don't go anywhere. I'll finish up here as fast as I can and then meet you there. I won't be long. We need to talk about this. And while you're waiting, say hi to Bobby for me, will you?"

Jon pulled the phone away from his ear and said, "Hey, Bobby, Karen says hi." Bobby blew Karen a kiss from the other side of the bar. Jon told Karen that he'd blown her the kiss.

"Blow him one back for me," she said.

"I don't think so."

"I'll be there in twenty minutes."

"Bye."

"Bye."

⋮    ⋮    ⋮

Forty-five minutes went by before Karen walked through the doorway. Afternoon sunlight outlined her figure through her skirt. She saw Bobby at the bar. "Hi, Bobby. Is Jon in here somewhere?" Bobby pointed toward Jon and then reached for a glass to pour another Redhook.

Jon stood to greet her. "Hi, Karen. Over here."

Karen asked Bobby, "Mind if we sit in a booth?"

"Be my guest. No doubt you two have a lot to talk about, with the witness-protection program and all. I'll bring your drinks."

"What did you tell him?" Karen asked Jon as they selected a booth near the back.

"Nothing that won't be in tomorrow's papers."

Carla piped up, saying, "That doctor's guilty as hell."

Bobby brought them their beers.

"You've had an interesting day," Karen said after they were alone. She reached for her beer and took a sip. "I've never heard of a U.S. marshal making a deal. FBI, maybe, but not a U.S. marshal. They don't do that. It's against their nature."

"Maybe they're just trying to close the book on a murdered witness."

"Could be," Karen said, "but I doubt it. I'll bet there's more to it than that. Carrie's left us with a few holes to fill in." She sipped on her beer.

Jon reached for his glass. "Yeah, I know. I've been working on that." He took a drink and then wiped the foam off his lip. "First there's Chester Dorsey. His killers knew that Carrie had called him, but they couldn't have known what was said. They tortured him to find out. They probably learned about Carrie's planned trip to Seattle, but she and Dorsey must not have set up a definitive date or time. If they had, he'd have told them about it."

"So we have a plausible motive for Chester's murder."

"Yeah, we do, but then there's Candy Peterson. What were they after there?"

A loud "Fuck you" came from the vicinity of the bar. Bobby and one of his regulars, Davie Wyman, were arguing about his state of inebriation.

"Offer him a free cup of coffee," Jon yelled from the booth. "And tell him to turn down the volume."

Davie yelled back at Jon to mind his own fucking business, saying that he didn't want any of Bobby's goddamned fucking too-strong black coffee.

"Watch your language," Carla injected from the other end of the bar. "What's a girl to think around here?"

Wyman leaned over toward Bobby and slurred a little too loudly in the general direction of his ear, "Yeah, well, we all know what that lying slut really thinks."

"Sycophant," she said under her breath as she focused back on her Manhattan. The noise level eventually died down as the toothless old rummy ran out of gas.

Jon continued, "You were about to say ..."

"We were talking about Candy Peterson," Karen said. "They obviously wanted to keep her from talking to you, but that doesn't explain the torture. They were after something else. And then there was Carrie's apartment. What were they looking for there?" Karen drained the rest of her beer.

"Want another one?" It was Bobby. He'd appeared at the side of their table. His inebriated customer was glowering at him from the corner of the bar. Carla Frehse was looking at them over her shoulder. She was again stirring her Manhattan with her finger. It was her third. Karen's glass was empty. Jon still had a little left in his.

"Sure, I'll have another."

Jon gulped the rest of his beer. "Make that two."

As Bobby left to get the drinks, Jon brought up the subject of the hospital digital tapes. "I keep thinking about them," he said. "I think the tapes are key. Somebody felt they were valuable enough to kill for."

"You don't know that," Karen answered. "They were stolen with the rest of Wolfson's records. Maybe it wasn't the tapes they were after at all. Maybe it was something else."

"Could be," he said, "but I don't think so. Those tapes contain a record of Wolfson's entire hospitalization. Maybe there's something there that explains his murder, or at least the search of Carrie's apartment."

"Too bad they were stolen," Karen said. "We'll never know what's on them now, not unless they're somehow recovered."

"Yeah, too bad."

"I have a theory about that." It was Bobby again. He brought the beers to the table and then sat down next to Karen. "Slide over," he said. "Make more room." She did. "Want to hear it?"

"Do I have a choice?"

Jon groaned. "He always has a theory."

"Yeah, well, maybe," Bobby answered. "And maybe you should talk a little less and listen a little more. You might learn something.

"But about those tapes, the ones you mentioned just a minute ago. If they're all that important, somebody would've had to have made copies, wouldn't they? Ms. Morse, your fancy-pants hospital administrator, wouldn't have set up her all-seeing AV system just to put her precious tapes in a public medical records room. You said in your article that it was installed specifically for Wolf, I mean Wolfson, and that he was the first patient to have been taped in such a way."

Karen and Jon looked at each other for a few moments. Jon then said to her, "He could have a point."

"Well, of course I have a point. Come on …"

Silence.

Bobby rolled his eyes. "COME ON …"

More silence.

"Jeez, you guys. Do I have to spell it out? If there are copies of those tapes lying around somewhere in Ocean City, why don't you go down there and get them? See for yourself if they're important or not."

"Come on, Bobby, you know we can't do that," Karen answered.

"Why not?" Bobby picked up Jon's beer and took a slug.

"Give me my beer back." He reached for his Redhook and took it back from Bobby.

"Well, first of all," Karen answered, "if there are copies, and we don't know that there are, they're a part of Wolfson's medical record. They're privileged. We can't touch them."

"Is that so?" Bobby said as he snuck another sip of Jon's beer.

"The hospital administrator, if she has them at all, isn't about to give them to us."

Bobby looked over at Jon and smirked, "Really?"

"So there's no way she's going to let us look at them. Case closed."

"Case closed? What's the matter with you guys?" Bobby drank

the rest of Jon's beer. "Do you want to see the tapes or not? Do I have to go down there and get them myself? How hard could it be? They've got to be locked up in the administrator's office. What's the big deal? It'd be a piece of cake."

Jon said to Karen, "He may have a point. I could call Mavis. She might be willing to help." He reached for her beer.

She pulled it back. "There probably aren't any tapes." She took a slug, then wiped her lip with the back of her index finger.

"Sure there are," Bobby answered. "There have to be."

Jon then said, "We're going to have to figure out a way to get them out of the hospital without anyone knowing about it."

"Jon," said Karen.

Jon ignored her. "How're we going to do that?" he asked Bobby. "It's hardly your piece of cake. There are bound to be problems."

"Oh, I'm sure you'll think of something," Bobby answered.

"Jon?" It was Karen again.

Bobby continued, "You always do—think of something, I mean." A sly smile worked its way across his face. Jon mimicked the smile.

"Jon, I don't like this." Karen's voice was stern.

Jon wiped the smile away. "Like what?"

"I don't at all like what you're thinking."

"What? You don't know what I'm thinking."

"Damn it, Jon, look at me." She pointed at her eyes with her fingers. "Taking those tapes is illegal; it's stealing. I can't have that. I'm a lieutenant on the Seattle police force, for Christ's sake. Don't listen to Bobby. He doesn't know what he's talking about."

Silence.

"Jon?"

# Chapter 27

JON SAT IN HIS Explorer in the Sisters of Mercy Medical Center parking lot. It was a gross understatement to say that he'd had an interesting day. His articles in the *Seattle Times* had created a sensation. They'd been picked up by the national wire services. He'd become an instant celebrity. Everyone wanted to schedule time with him, especially the radio and TV talk-show types. He'd turned them all down. He disliked punditry and pundits, and he wasn't about to allow himself to become just another talking head.

Karen had spent the morning meeting with Robbie. They rehashed what they'd learned about the Peterson and Dorsey murders, and in spite of all the new information about the witness-protection program, they didn't have much to go on. Karen brought up the subject of the Sisters of Mercy digital videotapes. Robbie thought that there was a good possibility that there were copies and that the tapes could potentially be important. But when he checked with the Ocean City Police Department, he was told that they didn't know anything about copies, and that if there were copies, they'd be strictly off limits. They'd already asked for

Stewart Wolf's medical records and had been stonewalled by the hospital. Alex Morse had turned them down and then had fought a subpoena on the basis of medical confidentiality. The police hadn't made a good enough case to overcome the confidentiality argument with a judge. "Somebody's trying to hide something," Robbie mused aloud.

Chap Alvord had called Jon at mid-morning to ask about Carrie and to remind him of their deal. "Call me anytime day or night," he'd said, "And, remember, I'll set the time and the place." Jon had assured him that he'd call, and then he'd called Karen to tell her that they needed to arrange the meeting. He'd reiterated that they needed to get their hands on the tapes. She'd said that she'd talk to Carrie about the meeting and then reaffirmed that he shouldn't do anything illegal.

Next he'd called Mavis. He'd told her that Carrie was well, safe, and in hiding. Then he'd asked her if she might know something about the possibility of digital videotape copies. She'd said that if there were copies, they'd be kept in Alex Morse's office, just as he'd guessed. She'd added that Alex usually left her office and the hospital for home somewhere between five and six in the evening, in case he was interested. Jon had replied that he was definitely interested. Mavis had told him that she was working a double shift and that the next shift change wasn't until eleven. She'd said that she could get a passkey that might get him into Alex's office, but she couldn't guarantee it. She'd give it to him in the hospital parking lot after her evening shift at eleven if he wished. She'd said that she was sorry she couldn't help him more, but that she couldn't afford to risk getting caught. She needed her job. He'd have to take it from there by himself. Jon thanked her, but he had no intention of taking it from there by himself. He'd immediately called Karen.

Karen answered after the first ring. "What? Are you crazy? No, no way, nope, not a chance in hell, not until hell freezes over!" She was emphatic. She wasn't going to go to Ocean City, and if she had anything to say about it, neither was he. "Do you understand just how much trouble you could get into doing something like that? What is it about 'nothing illegal' that you don't understand?"

Jon pleaded his case. He needed the tapes, and so did she. There had to be copies, and this was the only way to get them.

"We can't do this. If we can't get them legally, we can't get them, period. That's just the way it is."

Jon didn't answer.

"Jon … don't do this, Jon … . Jon, if you go down there and steal those tapes, I'll bust you myself. Grand theft, breaking and entering, obstruction of justice—I'll think of more. You'll mess up our case. We won't be able to use them in court if you take them illegally. Jon?"

After a moment's pause Jon answered, "Ocean City's just a little out of your jurisdiction, don't you think?" He had to pull the phone away from his ear when he heard her answer.

:    :    :

The lights in the parking lot were bright but widely spaced, and he'd had no trouble finding a parking space that was well shadowed. He watched the last of the graveyard shift as they parked their cars all around him. It was 10:50. Clouds were hanging low, and an enveloping mist condensed on his windows. He waited. He shivered. "Mavis, where are you?" Several people walked out the front door. They were followed a few seconds later by a few more. Then a steady stream of people moved from the hospital entrance toward the parking lot. Jon sat forward in his seat. He searched the crowd.

Cars started, lights flashed on, and people started driving away. Jon looked at his watch. It was five past eleven. The flow of people increased. Another twenty minutes passed before he finally spotted her. She stood just inside the hospital's entrance.

Jon got out of the car and walked across the parking lot. Mavis greeted him by the doorway, her hands on her ample hips. "You ready for this?" she asked.

"Why, what's the matter?"

"There's been a change of plans." She waited for several stragglers to clear the entrance before she continued. "OK, I've got the key; it's a passkey. With any luck it'll open the door to her office." She reached into her purse, retrieved the passkey, and handed it to Jon. "Throw it away when you're done with it. I got it out of maintenance, and they aren't numbered. They'll never miss it.

"You know where the office is; you've been there before. There are two doors, an outer door to the waiting room and an inner door to Ms. Morse's office. Cross your fingers that the key will open both. The tapes, if they're anywhere, will be in there somewhere. Once inside, you'll have to find them on your own.

"Security will check on the office every hour or so. They'll check the outer door to make sure it's locked, and they might shine a flashlight through the door's window to check the waiting room, but they won't come inside. As long as you're quiet and they can't see any light, you should be all right. Do you have a flashlight?"

Jon pulled a small flashlight out of his pocket and clicked it on and off.

"Good. Now about the change in plans. I'm coming with you, at least to the outer office."

Jon wrinkled his forehead. "What?" His eyebrows pinched together.

"There's a new guy at the information desk, Officer Crumpacker. He works nights. They replaced the volunteer with a security guard. He's not too bright, but he'll do his job. He'll check your ID and ask you to sign in unless you're with me. There's no other way to do this. You don't want to have your name on a registry on the same night as a break-in. It'd document your presence in the hospital."

Jon shook his head. "Mavis, what if we get caught? I might get a slap on the wrist, a misdemeanor breaking-and-entering or trespass, but you'd get fired. I can't let that happen."

"We won't get caught," she said. "That's why I'm doing this. It's now a two-person job. I'll get you in and watch your back."

"Yeah, but what if I have to mess up the place a little?" He looked into her eyes. "Even if I don't have to mess it up, I'm going to take the tapes. Sooner or later they'll discover that they're missing. I don't want them to be able to connect you with this thing."

Mavis chuckled. "Don't you worry about me. I can take care of myself. You just be sure to take care of your own self. And do me a favor, will you? Find something on those tapes that'll help Carrie."

"I'll do my best," he answered. "Is there anything else I need to know about that guy Crumpacker, or security in general, before we start?"

"I don't think so. As I said, he's not too bright. That should be it."

"Then thanks, Mavis." He held the key up in the air. "Let's do it."

"Don't mention it." She put her hand on his arm. "And I really mean that. Don't *ever* mention it." She chuckled again and smiled a broad smile. Jon nodded his head, and they started into the lobby.

:　:　:

The hospital lobby was well lit and nearly empty. The shift change was all but complete. Jim Crumpacker, the security guard, was sitting at the information desk just where Mavis had said he would be. His eyes shifted back and forth from the lobby to a *Penthouse* magazine that he kept half-hidden below desk level in his lap. He paid no attention as Jon and Mavis walked past. A young-looking janitor was sweeping the floor. Newspaper vending machines were still partially filled with now almost day-old newspapers. Jon could clearly see his headline through the window in the *Seattle Times* box. The air smelled of a hospital. They turned down a hallway toward the offices of the hospital administrator. Their footsteps echoed off the hard-surfaced walls and floor.

The door to Alex Morse's office was located halfway down the corridor on the right. They could see that it was dark inside. Jon took out the passkey. "Here, put these on before you touch anything," Mavis said. She handed him a pair of surgical latex gloves and then put on a pair herself. "You can't be too careful."

Jon tried the key in the lock. It unlocked with a click. They opened the door and quickly went inside. Mavis closed the door and checked to be sure that it was relocked before they proceeded to the inner door.

"Is everything clear?" Jon half-whispered.

Mavis looked out through the window into the hallway and down toward the lobby. "It looks OK to me," she whispered back.

Jon inserted the key into the inner door lock. He tried to turn it to the right. It wouldn't turn. He jiggled the key in the lock. Nothing happened. He tried forcing the key to turn. Nothing happened.

Mavis whispered, "What's wrong?"

"The key won't turn. She must have a special lock for her inner sanctum." He tried it once more. "We're going to have to break it. Do you want to leave? This is going to make a little noise."

"No, too late to back out now, but thanks for the thought. Hold on a second." She went back over to the window and again checked the corridor. It was clear. "OK, go ahead, but be careful with the noise."

The first time Jon hit the door with his shoulder, it held fast. He rubbed his shoulder, sheepishly looking back at Mavis, and then he shrugged. Mavis shook her head. Then he hit it again, harder this time; still it wouldn't give. Mavis rolled her eyes. Then she moved over next to him. "Move out of the way." She rammed it herself, using her bulk like a linebacker. There was a loud crack. The doorjamb splintered, and the door flung open. Jon's jaw dropped, along with his self-esteem. "Somebody sure as hell heard that," she said. "How bad is the door?"

"Not good," Jon answered. "They might miss seeing the damage in the dark, but if they hit it with their flashlight beams …"

"OK, look. You go inside and look for the tapes. I'll hang out down there in the waiting room by the couches in the shadows."

"And if the security guard comes?"

"He probably won't, but if he does, I'll take care of it."

"You're sure?"

"I said I'll take care of it. Now go on."

Jon went inside and closed the door behind him.

:   :   :

Jon took out his flashlight and turned it on. Alex Morse's office was just as he remembered it. He first went to the desk. It wasn't locked. He opened and rummaged through all seven of its drawers. The tapes weren't there. Then he went over to the wooden file cabinets against the wall. There were four of them, and they were all locked. He tried popping the locks with his penknife, and when that didn't work, he picked up a steel-bladed letter opener from the desk and pried the locks open one by one. The wood split apart each time he pried open a drawer. The tapes weren't in any of them.

He shone his flashlight around the room. He worried that Alex might have locked them up in a safe somewhere, or maybe there weren't any tapes. He was looking at some shelves when he heard a noise from outside. He froze in place.

:   :   :

Mavis saw the security guards through the window in the door. There were two of them, and they didn't seem to be in a hurry. They were talking about the Portland Trailblazers. She crouched down in a corner by the couches. They were saying something about Paul Allen moving the team to a larger market.

The guards approached the door. The doorknob rattled. One of the guards knocked on the glass with his knuckles. The other turned on his flashlight and shone it through the window.

Mavis pressed herself against the wall. She took a deep breath and held it.

The flashlight beam danced across the secretary's desk, across the door to Alex's inner office, down the wall, and then onto the couches in the waiting area.

When the beam started to retrace its path, Mavis was sure that they must have seen the ruined door lock and doorjamb, but the guards continued their conversation, and then the beam flicked off. Finally they turned around and started back toward the lobby.

As their footsteps died away, Mavis let out her breath. She moved toward the inner office door. "That was close," she whispered to Jon as she crept inside. Jon's flashlight was off. She turned hers on. "Find anything yet?"

"Not yet," Jon whispered back. "They're not in the desk or in the file cabinets. I busted up the locks on the file cabinets pretty good."

Mavis shone her light on the files. "I can see that," she said. Her light scanned the room. "What are these?" She was illuminating something on a bookshelf right behind him.

Jon turned around. He saw a row of nine plastic containers neatly lined up on the shelf. They looked like they could be digital tape containers. He pulled one down and opened it. "Well, what do you know? Bobby was right."

"They were right behind you," she said. "I'll bet you can't find the butter in the refrigerator, either."

Jon pulled a folded plastic garbage bag out of his pocket and opened it. Together they put the tapes inside. Then they took off their gloves, tossed them in the bag, folded the extra plastic over the tapes, and, careful not to touch anything with their bare hands, left the office.

Mavis checked the hallway before they left the outer door; it looked clear. Then, just as they stepped outside, a voice said sharply, "All right, you cocksuckers, hold it right there." The voice came from somewhere behind them.

Jon froze.

"You, fuck face, what's in the bag?" It was a female voice.

Jon braced himself, getting ready to run. Mavis put her hand on his arm.

"Jean?" Mavis turned around toward the source of the voice. "Jean, is that you? What are you doing out here?" She gave her a stern nurse look. "Shouldn't you be up in your room?" She leaned toward Jon and said out of the side of her mouth, "It's Jean Reseburg, Tourette's syndrome. She gets out and does this every now and then."

Reseburg pointed at Jon. "Who's the monkey cunt?" She twitched the left side of her face and continuously blinked as she spoke.

Mavis cut her off. "Come on, Jean. Let's go back to your room. I'll go up with you." Then she whispered to Jon, "Get out of here."

Jon started to walk. He cautiously carried his bundle down the hall toward the lobby.

"Piss, shit, assholes!"

Jon turned the corner and moved toward the front door. He

glanced at the security guard as he walked by. Crumpacker was engrossed in his *Penthouse* magazine. He didn't even bother to look up.

# Chapter 28

Jon drove home to an empty house. The sun would be up in a few hours. Leon greeted him at the door. Karen did not. She'd walked out after he'd told her that he was leaving for Ocean City. They'd had one of the worst arguments of their relationship. A note tacked to his pillow read, "**THIEF.**" It was underlined three times. He ripped it off, fell into bed, and immediately fell into an almost comatose sleep.

When his alarm rang at 7:30, he rolled over to see Leon sleeping next to him in Karen's spot. He hit the alarm and then checked it to make sure that he'd turned it all the way off and not just put it on snooze. Then he called his office to tell them that he wouldn't be in until later in the day, and finally he pulled the covers up over his head and went back to sleep. After what seemed like only a few seconds but was really almost half an hour, he felt the covers slowly slide away from his face. He started to wake. An ice-cold something splashed onto and over his skin. His eyes popped open. Karen was standing next to his bed, dressed in running clothes. Her arm was extended over his head, and her hand was holding a large glass in an almost horizontal position. A stream of water connected the glass to the tip of his nose.

"Jesus Christ!" He bolted upright. He flailed. His feet kicked at the covers. He jolted to the side in a ball of blankets and sheets, and then he rolled off the bed and bounced onto the floor.

Leon looked over at Karen with surprised eyes. He was still in her spot. "What are you looking at?" she said to him. "You're just as bad as he is." She tossed what water she had left in her glass onto the dog. He jumped off the bed and ran into the kitchen.

Karen then shifted her fiery focus back to Jon. "You're an idiot, you know that?" She eyed him as he got up from the floor. He unwrapped the covers and sheets from around his body and put them back onto the bed. "You think this is funny, don't you? How can you expect us to live together when you … ."

"Karen."

"What?" They stared at each other without speaking for a few seconds. "You're such a moron. You stole those tapes; I know you did. I've been sleeping with a moron!"

"A moron?" Jon cracked a smile. He couldn't help it.

"Wipe that smile off your face."

"Come on, Karen. No harm's been done."

"No harm done? Damn it, Jon, why do you do these things?" Karen crossed her arms. Leon peeked into the room from around the corner. "What am I supposed to do when they figure out what you were doing down there? You probably left your fingerprints all over the place."

"No, I didn't." They stood there for a moment, again staring at each other.

"Somebody probably recognized you."

"Unlikely," he answered. They continued their staring contest.

"You do have the tapes, don't you?" she finally asked. "There were copies, weren't there? That's what you drove all the way down there to get!"

"I have them," he said. He paused, then continued, "But who says I stole them? Maybe I found them. Maybe someone gave them to me. I'd love to tell you about it, but it would be unethical for me to reveal my sources." He wiggled his eyebrows up and down.

"Damn it, Jon."

"You already said that."

"Aghhh!" Karen's face flushed. She tossed the glass at him. He tried to dodge. It bounced off his side onto the bed. He picked it up and turned back to face her.

"Come on, Karen. What's the big deal?"

"What's the big deal? You know very well what the big deal is. You could be prosecuted for this."

There was another long pause. Then Jon said, "The newspaper will back me up; you know they will. They have an excellent legal department. No one's going to nail me for stealing the tapes. And since their source is unknown, we won't have to worry about the chain of evidence."

She just stared at him.

"You know it's true."

Another pause. "Damn it, Jon," she finally said for the third time. " Of course I know it's true! And of course you'll get away with it; you always do. That's what pisses me off so much." She kicked at the covers.

"It was the only way." He ran his hands through his hair, brushing the water away.

"It's never the only way," Karen insisted. "Someday you're going to get into real trouble. And when you do I'll ..."

"Look, Karen, I know you think this is just about a newspaper story, but it's not. And it's not about the SPD and your Peterson and Dorsey investigations, either. It's about Carrie and trying to clear her name. It's about trying to find out if she's playing straight with us. Do you want to look at the tapes?" He picked the wad of covers off the floor and then started separating the sheets from the blankets.

"Of course I want to look at them, but ..."

"OK, then, are you sorry you poured that water on me?"

"Damn it, Jon."

"I think that's the fourth time you said that."

∶　　∶　　∶

Jon connected the digital tape player to his television set and pushed the first tape into its slot. Then he pushed the play button. An image of a man lying in a hospital bed came up on the TV screen. He didn't move. The date and time were enumerated in the lower right-hand corner. Alex Morse was in the room, along with someone else they didn't recognize. Alex asked if the equipment was working. The other man said that it was. He approached the camera, the image jiggled a little, and then they left. Time elapsed, and then an intern came in and performed a physical exam. Nurses, including Candy Peterson, came in on several occasions, sometimes doing something with the IV. Peterson had several of what seemed to be one-sided conversations with her patient, speaking softly to him while she worked. Wolfson sometimes answered with what sounded like garbled words, but most of the time he did not answer. After forty-five minutes Karen said, "This is taking too long. Let's fast-forward through the parts when nothing's happening." Karen ejected the first tape after it finished, and Jon left to let Leon out into the backyard. He returned in time for the start of the second.

Carrie Williams made her first appearance on the second tape. She came into the room alone, introduced herself to her patient, and asked a few basic mental-status questions such as, "Do you know where you are? What day is it? Do you know what month it is?" And then she started her neurological examination. Wolfson didn't seem to hear, and he didn't answer. He hardly moved at all. Candy Peterson entered again just as she was finishing. She greeted Carrie, adjusted the flow rate on the IV, hung a new plastic bag full of clear fluid on the IV pole, asked Carrie about Wolfson's prognosis, and then asked how much time he had left. Karen paused the tape just as Peterson turned away from her patient to leave. "Jon, did you see that?"

"What?"

She rewound the tape and played it again. "There." She stopped the tape again. "That." Jon focused on the tape.

Wolfson had opened his eyes. He looked at Peterson and tracked her as she moved around his bed. Neither Carrie nor Peterson had seemed to notice. "He's awake," Jon said, "And he's not nearly as out of it as he makes out to be." Wolfson shut his eyes again after Peterson turned away. Karen restarted the tape. Carrie finished her physical exam and then followed Peterson out of the room. That was the end of the second tape.

Nothing much happened on the third and fourth tapes.

The fifth again started with an unmoving Frankie Wolfson lying in his hospital bed. Every time someone entered the room, Karen would slow the tape to see who it was—more often than not it was Candy Peterson—and to check Wolfson's reaction;

there was none. They'd listen to what was said and watch what was done, and then Karen would speed the tape up again. They went almost all the way through the tape before Carrie came into the room again. A shorter man was with her, and he was carrying a hospital chart.

The man with Carrie identified himself as Joe Unis. He was an intern, and he was talking to Carrie about the man that they called Stewart Wolf. He was going over his medical history. "… severe case of squash rot, glioblastoma, grade four, with lots of necrosis. According to the chart he's been circling the drain for about a week. He's admitted for terminal care."

"Nice, Joe," she said to her intern. "Let's hold down the 'squash rot' and 'circling the drain' comments in front of our patients, shall we? He might've heard you." Then she took a penlight out of her pocket and shone it in Wolfson's eyes to check his pupilary reflexes. She pinched his fingernails, uncovered his feet, and scratched his soles with the back of a reflex hammer. When she asked Wolfson if he knew his name, if he knew where he was, and if he knew what month it was, he mumbled incoherent nothings in response. She then told Unis that Wolfson was oversedated and that he should check his meds. She asked him to cut back on the sedation.

Next she listened to Wolfson's heart, rolled him on his side and listened to his lungs, and palpated his abdomen. She checked for enlarged lymph nodes in his neck, under his arms, and in his groin. She checked his catheter and the amount of urine in his catheter bag. Finally she took the chart from her intern, wrote some notes, and started out of the room.

"What do you think?" Unis asked.

Carrie answered quietly so that her patient couldn't hear.

The recorder didn't pick it up. She said something about Unis coming back to do a complete H and P as they walked through the doorway.

Jon reached for the remote control and stopped the tape. He looked at Karen. "That wasn't much."

"What's an H and P?"

"A history and physical exam, I think."

"Start it up again. Let's keep going."

Jon pushed the play button, sped up the tape, ejected it when it finished, and put in another one. It was a while before Carrie returned. She walked into the room without speaking, took out her flashlight, shined it in her patient's eyes, and then adjusted something on the IV flow pump. She gently patted him on the shoulder before she left. Sometime later, near the end of the tape, she entered the room again. This time she walked directly over to the digital tape recorder, and the image on the tape jiggled a little. Jon could see her mouth something, but he couldn't make out what it was. Then the sound went dead.

"She turned off the sound! Why would she do that?"

Carrie pulled a small syringe out of her pocket as she moved over to the IV stand. She twisted the plastic cap off the needle attached to the end of the syringe and injected a small amount of clear fluid through a rubber stop-cap into the IV tubing. Then she pulled a chair over adjacent to the head of her patient's bed and said something. She sat down, patted him on the shoulder again, and waited.

A minute or so later, Wolfson started to move. Carrie put her face close to her patient's ear. She started to talk. She turned her back, clearly blocking the camera's view of her lips. Jon couldn't tell what she was saying, so he focused his attention on Wolfson.

At times it looked as if Wolfson were listening. His eyes would seem to clear, and sometimes his lips would move in response to something that she'd said. At others he appeared unresponsive. Then she turned around, glanced at the camera, and moved the position of her head, deliberately shielding his face from view. Carrie sat there with him for almost twenty minutes.

At one point Wolfson made a kind of beckoning movement with his hand, and Carrie responded by leaning over and placing her ear very close to his lips. Then she abruptly pulled her head back and shook it as if saying no. From that point on he remained almost inanimate.

Carrie finally stood up and moved her chair back to the place where she'd gotten it. She turned the sound back on. Jon could hear her footsteps echo off the walls as she walked out of the room. He paused the tape.

"What was that all about?" Karen asked. "Why turn off the sound, and what did she put in the IV?"

"It seemed to wake him up," Jon said. "They were having a conversation about something. They may've been talking about assisted suicide, but maybe it was something else. She deliberately blocked the camera so we couldn't use a lip reader."

"It was definitely something else. There was something going on there, something important. Call it intuition, but there was definitely something going on. Why would he whisper in her ear like that? What could he have said?"

"There's only one way to find out," Jon answered. "We ask her."

"Uh-huh, but what's this 'we' stuff?" This time it was Karen who wiggled her eyebrows up and down at Jon. "This is police business, Jon. I'll do the interrogating here. You're out of the loop, remember?"

The last person to enter the room was Candy Peterson. As she walked over to see Wolfson, he seemed to beckon her closer. Then he appeared to say something that they couldn't hear. Jon replayed the segment and turned up the volume, but they still couldn't hear what was said. Then he played the rest of the tape, ejected it, and inserted the last one.

Carrie was next seen walking into the room with a plastic IV bag filled with clear fluid. She hung the bag on Wolfson's IV pole and then connected it to his flow pump with a length of clear, coiled IV tubing. Next she adjusted the pump, patted him on the shoulder, quietly said something that sounded like "Are you sure?" and then waited for a response. She got none. Finally she said, "Goodnight, Stewart," and then walked back out of the room.

"That's where she turned up the morphine," Karen said.

"Yeah, I think so."

They watched Wolfson as he lay immobile on his bed for a few seconds, and then they sped up the tape to the point where the nurses rushed into the room to start the resuscitation effort. At that point Jon slowed it back down to normal speed.

Jon and Karen watched Wolfson die. The cardiac-arrest code played out to its conclusion. Then the real Dr. Bennett entered the room and questioned Carrie. An argument ensued. They watched until all the players left. Finally two orderlies came to take the body away to the morgue. Then Jon pushed the pause button. "I guess that's it." He glanced at Karen before reanimating the picture. Sometime later a technician came in and turned off the recorder.

# Chapter 29

JON SHUT OFF the tape player. "We've got to contact Carrie. You can ask her about her conversation with Wolfson. I'll stay out of it, but I need to arrange her meeting with Alvord. I made a deal, and something tells me that he has all kinds of ways of making me stick to it."

"I'm sure he does, and you bet you'll stay out of it." Karen made the call. The policewoman staying with Carrie answered and then called her to the phone. Karen explained about Jon's meeting with Alvord and then about his deal.

"He had no right to do that," Carrie answered. "I'm not meeting with anybody."

She told her that Stewart Wolf was really Frankie Wolfson, a protected witness, then explained about the Grinstein syndicate, the Medicare scam, and Wolfson's stolen money. "I think it's important that you meet with the marshals," she said. "Those Grinstein syndicate people are ruthless. They've already killed four people, and they won't hesitate to do it again. They'll track you down unless we stop them; it's for your own good."

"Thanks for the advice, but I don't think so."

"I'll go with you." She told her about the digital tapes.

"You have copies of the tapes? You've seen them?"

Karen said that she had.

"May I see them?"

There was a pause. "I don't see why not. There's a segment on there where you turned off the sound. Why did you do that? It looked to me like you were having a real two-sided conversation with your patient. What were you talking about, and why didn't you want it recorded on tape?"

"We were talking about his death," Carrie said. "It's a very private and personal matter."

"That's it?" Karen asked. "Nothing else?"

"Nothing else. I gave him a stimulant so we could discuss it. I wanted to be sure I was doing the right thing."

"And if we show you the tapes, you'll meet with the marshals?"

Another pause. Finally she said, "All right, I'll meet with Marshal Alvord. And then she added, "But you needn't come along. As a matter of fact, I don't want you to come along. It's not that I don't trust you; I just don't know you. I do trust Jon. I'll go with him. And as a condition I want to see the tapes before I go, all of them." She returned the phone to the policewoman who was staying with her.

Karen talked with the policewoman and made arrangements for Carrie to view the tapes. Then she hung up.

"She wants to see the tapes," she said to Jon. "It's a condition for meeting with Alvord. I'm having her brought over to view them.

"There's something there, something on the tapes. I can feel it. It's something that she's concerned about. If we watch her closely while she's watching the tapes, maybe we can figure it out.

"Oh, and, by the way, you're back in it. She won't go see the marshals with me. She'll only go with you. She trusts you and only you for some stupid reason or other."

"Uh-huh," Jon answered. "Doesn't everybody?"

Jon made the call to Alvord, who answered after the first ring. The entire conversation took only a few minutes. Carrie was to meet with the marshals at a safe house an hour east of town near Snoqualmie Falls. The meeting was set for 4:00 PM that afternoon. Jon would drive her there, and he could attend the meeting if he wished. They would meet for approximately two hours, and then that would be the end of it. Witness-protection services would not be available to Carrie.

Carrie arrived at Jon's house with her policewoman escort, and then she watched the tapes, all of them. She replayed a few segments but made no comments one way or the other on what she saw. Karen noticed nothing unusual with her body language. She asked her again about turning off the sound, and she got the same answer. Carrie said it was for her patient's privacy. It was a plausible explanation, and Karen decided not to push it.

At 1:00 Carrie climbed into Jon's Explorer to leave for her meeting with Alvord. She was expecting to be questioned, but she had a few questions of her own for the marshals. They drove out of his garage, down Madison Avenue, and then over to the interstate. Traffic was light, and they quickly got ahead of their schedule. They'd originally planned for a lunch stop, possibly in Issaquah, but neither one of them was really very hungry, so instead of stopping, they drove all the way east to the Preston exit, where they joined the Preston–Falls City road. They reached Falls City at 1:37 PM.

"Carrie, would you take a look at this?" Jon said. He handed her a folded scrap of notepaper. "They're Alvord's directions to the safe house."

Carrie unfolded the paper, then squinted. "Your handwriting's terrible. You should've been a doctor." She read the directions. "It says to follow the highway out of Falls City toward North Bend."

"We're doing that," Jon said.

"The river's supposed to be on our right."

"It's there." He nodded his head toward the river.

"When you reach a fish hatchery, there should be a sign. Look out for a gravel road on the left. It's the first one after the hatchery, and you should see it just after we start up a steep hill."

After driving for a few minutes, Carrie said, "There's the fish hatchery. The falls are just up the hill." A few minutes later she said, "There's the gravel road. Turn left on the road and follow it for 1.7 miles." Jon turned onto the road and checked his odometer. "And at 1.7 miles turn right."

Jon followed the old logging road as it twisted in and out through third-growth forest. It was only loosely covered with gravel and was still heavily rutted from last winter's rains. The going was slow, even in the Explorer, and it took almost eight minutes to traverse the short distance. But even at that speed they almost missed the next turn. That road was hardly a road at all; it was more of a path: two shale-covered tire tracks winding through the trees, separated by some low-standing grass and moss.

Jon shifted into four-wheel drive. "Where does it say to go from here?"

"Have we gone 1.7 miles yet?" Jon nodded yes. "Then turn right. That's all it says."

Jon followed the road. The road bumped and twisted up a hill through thickening trees until finally, after approximately half a mile, it opened into a clearing several acres in area. It looked as if it had been logged out at least half a century ago. Most of the tree stumps had been removed, and the plants of the forest floor had been replaced by a meandering meadow. An occasional wildflower was still in bloom.

A large log house was sitting at the apex of the clearing. It looked solid, and it looked old. Its position gave it a clear and commanding view in all directions. It would be very difficult for anyone to approach the house without being seen.

The twin tire tracks that defined a facsimile of a road led to a newer log-construction outbuilding adjacent to the house. It was large enough to hold three or four vehicles, possibly even some heavy equipment. There were no other buildings in the clearing.

Jon glanced at Carrie. "It looks like we've arrived." They followed the road to its end.

Jon checked his watch when he stepped out of the car; it was 1:53 PM. They were two hours early. His was the only car in the drive or on the property, as far as he could tell.

He walked over to the outbuilding and looked through its garage door window. It was dark inside, and although he could see only the area directly behind the door, it looked empty. He tried the door. It was locked.

Carrie had moved over toward the house. It had a large eighteen-foot-wide porch surrounding it on all sides. Its thick and solid front door was fronted on the outside by an old-fashioned screened door. All the windows were screened as well.

She knocked on the door. There was no answer. She tried the doorknob. It was locked. She knocked again.

Jon joined her on the porch. "I'll go check around back," he said. He disappeared around the side of the house. The back door and all of the windows were also locked.

Carrie sat down on an old wooden porch swing hanging from two chains bolted into the roof of the porch. When Jon returned from the other side of the house, she invited him to join her. "You might as well have a seat," she said. She patted the wooden slats beside her. "We're going to be waiting here for a while."

Jon looked at his watch. It was 2:02 PM. "In a minute," he said. Instead, he went over to the front door and slid his fingers over the top of the doorjamb. There was nothing there but dust. He looked under the mud-stained doormat and then under an empty clay pot sitting on the porch to the left of the door.

"What are you doing?" Carrie asked. She was pumping the swing with her legs.

"I'm looking for a key."

"Come on, Jon. This is a safe house. There aren't going to be any keys lying around." She let the swing settle into a gentle oscillation.

"You never know," he said as he continued to search the area near the front door.

Carrie shut her eyes and started to hum. She was humming George Gershwin's "Summertime," trying to forget about why they were there, when she heard, "Oh, yeah!"

She snapped her brain back into the present. "What?"

"And you said they wouldn't leave a key at a safe house." He held up a copper key he'd found in a plastic baggie under the front steps.

"Well, well, what do you know?" She eyed the key. "Maybe this safe house isn't so safe after all."

Jon tried the key in the front door lock. The lock turned. The door opened. Carrie hopped off her swing and stepped inside the screen door. "Hello? Is anybody in here?" After waiting a moment and hearing no answer, they went inside.

There was a large front room furnished in lodge-style furniture, with two couches and several chairs facing a large stone fireplace. It had a high ceiling, and the walls were log. There were several Navaho-style rugs on the floor. The room connected with a dining room containing a round pine table surrounded by eight chairs. The updated kitchen was just beyond that. Carrie walked back through the dining room to the far side of the living room. A solid-looking heavy pine door was closed and locked. There were no outside windows in that corner of the house, and the area had a faint musty smell. She asked Jon to try his key. It didn't fit the lock, and the lock wouldn't turn, so they moved on. They finished their exploration of the first floor and then moved up the stairs to the second.

The second floor was all bedrooms and bathrooms. There were four bedrooms and two bathrooms off a central hallway around the east, north, and west sides of the house, and a larger master bedroom with its own bath on the south. The windows in the master bedroom had a view of the approaching road all the way down to the trees. Jon looked down at his car and then at his watch. It was 2:19 PM. "They won't be here for at least another hour."

Carrie also looked at her watch. She confirmed the time. "We could go up to North Bend and get something to eat if you're hungry. We could kill some time there."

"No, thanks," Jon answered. "I'm not even close to hungry. Karen and I went out to the Ewe Club last night, and I'm still working on Chef Tom's lamb. It's the best lamb in the state; Chef Tom is a maestro. I just want to get through this."

"Me, too," she said. "It'd just be something to do." She sat down on a wooden bench next to the window so she could see down the road. "I guess we just sit around and wait." She leaned against the wall. "I should've brought a book."

There was a slat-back chair at a desk in a corner away from the window. Jon pulled the chair over near Carrie's bench and joined her there. He paused a moment before saying, "Carrie, there's something I wanted to talk to you about this morning, but I never got the chance." He settled into his chair. "I've been doing a little research into Wolfson's money-laundering operation." He waited for a response, and when she offered none, he went on. "According to court records the feds have traced some of his money from the Bahamas to the Cayman Islands and then on to South Africa, to Switzerland, and then back to Curacao in the Dutch Antilles in the Caribbean. Apparently he set up a group of Dutch companies to receive the cash and then transferred ownership of their shares to corporations in Lichtenstein." He leaned forward just a bit. "You wouldn't know anything about any of that, would you?"

Carrie tilted her head to the side and looked crossways at Jon. "Is this what the marshals want to talk to me about?"

Jon answered, "I don't know. Lichtenstein is the only country in the world that issues bearer stock certificates. They're as good as cash. You set up a corporation, you dump a bunch of assets into its corporate account, and then you have stock certificates made out to 'bearer.' Anyone holding the corporate stock certificates can anonymously exchange them at any one of a number of international financial institutions for the assets held by the corporations. And when the assets are all cash ..."

"It sounds like a money launderer's dream come true," Carrie said.

"Yes, it does, doesn't it? And Wolfson, of course, was a money launderer. He was the only one who knew the names of the corporations. The feds have run into a dead end." Jon pulled his chair a bit closer.

"Wolfson stashed about a hundred million dollars' worth of those Lichtenstein bearer shares out there somewhere. That's the money he ripped off from the Grinstein crime syndicate." Jon paused and then shifted his weight. "Carrie, when you had that conversation with Wolfson in the hospital, the one we saw on tape when you turned off the sound ..."

"Yes?"

"Well, did he tell you anything about ..."

Carrie interrupted him. "You think I'm a thief?"

He answered quickly. "No."

"You think Wolfson told me where his money is."

"Carrie, it doesn't matter what I think. It's those other guys from the Grinstein syndicate, the ones that killed Candy Peterson and Chester Dorsey—they're the ones I'd be worrying about if I were you, not me. And, remember, they've seen the tapes, too. They killed Linda the medical records clerk to get them."

He was about to say something else when he noticed a gray Ford 500 break out from the trees. He stood to get a better look out the window. He checked his watch; it was 2:41 PM. It slowly drove up the driveway and stopped behind his Explorer. A man and a woman got out. Jon could clearly see their faces. "It's the marshals," he said. "Chap Alvord and somebody else. They're early. I guess we won't have to sit here and wait around all afternoon after all." He turned his head toward Carrie.

Carrie too was looking out the window. Her eyes were wide; her jaw had dropped. "Oh, God, no! No, please, no!" She grabbed Jon around the biceps with her left hand. She felt her heart thump in her chest. She turned away from the window and frantically looked around the bedroom.

"Carrie, what is it? What's the matter?"

She stared at him for an instant, and then blurted, "Those marshals!" Her throat was dry. Her voice was hoarse. "They're not who you think they are." She was breathing fast. She could barely talk. "That's Dr. Bennett, and the woman—she's the one who played Stewart Wolf's wife." She squeezed Jon's arm so tight that it hurt. "They're not here to talk." She swallowed hard. "They're here to kill us!" Her eyes flashed toward the doorway. "We've got to get out of here. We've got to get out of here now! We've got to find a place to hide!"

# Chapter 30

THE FIRST THING U.S. Marshals Chap Alvord and Ana Chestnut noticed when they cleared the trees was the black Explorer parked in front of the outbuilding.

"They beat us," Chestnut said.

"It doesn't matter," Alvord answered. "We can deal with it. It might even save us some time."

They pulled to a stop behind Jon's car and got out.

Chestnut walked over to the Explorer, looked inside, and then scanned the clearing. "Do you see anyone?"

Alvord joined her. "No," he said, looking around the clearing, "I don't." He walked over to the outbuilding and checked the lock on the door. It was still locked. He walked around its periphery, and when he returned, he said, "There's nobody back there. They may've found the key under the porch. My guess is that they're inside."

"Yeah, well, let's hope so," she answered. "We don't want to screw this up."

"No screw-ups," Alvord said as he pulled his gun out of the holster attached to his belt. He checked it over, ejected the clip, checked the clip to make sure it was full, reinserted it, and put it back in its holster. The firing chamber was empty. He left his coat unbuttoned and open. "Let's try not to make a mess, shall we?" He started toward the house.

Chestnut left her gun in her purse and walked with him to the front door. It was unlocked. They opened the door and stepped inside. There was no sign of Jon or Carrie.

Alvord called, "Hello?"

No answer.

"Carrie? Jon? Are you guys in here?"

No answer.

Beams of afternoon sunlight streamed in through the windows. Suspended particles of dust hung illuminated in the air. They smelled the faint musty smell. There was nothing but quiet. Nothing moved. The room looked as if it hadn't been disturbed in some time.

They scanned the area. Alvord went left and Chestnut went right. Alvord tried the door to the electronics room; it was still locked. Then Chestnut saw a single partial footprint in the dust on the floor. She whispered, "They're here." She pointed to Alvord and then motioned toward the dining room and kitchen, indicating that he should check them out. Then she pointed to herself and then to the stairs.

She walked to the stairway, glanced at Alvord, and then, sending her voice up to the second floor, said, "Carrie? Jon? Are you up there?"

No answer.

She reached into her handbag and removed a standard Justice Department-issue ten-millimeter Glock. She chambered a round. "OK," she said to Alvord, "let's find them." She started up the stairs.

# Chapter 31

JON WATCHED THE two marshals get out of their car. Carrie jerked on his arm. "They're going to try to kill us! Come on! Let's get out of here! We've got to get away!"

"We'll never make it," he answered. "Not downstairs. They'll get us before we get to the back door. We've got to find another way out."

Carrie ran toward the bedroom door. "Come on!"

Jon followed, trying to be quiet. Carrie didn't care about the noise. She ran into the hall and then banged open the door to the bedroom farthest away from the front of the house. It was as far away from the front door as she could get.

She went straight for a back window, opened it and pushed out the screen. She looked down. It was way too far for her to jump, but she saw another possibility. The window was about four feet away from the corner of the house, where its intersecting notched- log construction formed a kind of natural ladder. If she could make it over there, it would be easy to climb down.

Jon joined her at the window. He stuck his head out. She pointed out the crossing logs. "I think we can make it," he said. Distant voices floated up the stairs.

"Hello? Carrie? Jon? Are you guys in here?"

"Shit!"

Jon swung his leg over the sill and climbed out the window. Then he eased himself down the wall to the point where he was hanging on to the sill by his hands. His legs were dangling.

"Jon, be careful," Carrie whispered. "And hurry up."

He swung his legs over toward the corner of the house. He missed.

"Shit!"

He looked down at the ground. He inched his hands over toward the very left corner of the windowsill and tried again. This time his feet touched, and he hooked them around the crossed logs. He let go of the sill with his left hand and reached for the corner while still hanging by his right. His feet were on the logs. He stretched and then grabbed on to a notched log end, pulling himself over to where he could stand upright. After he shifted his weight to his feet, he looked over at Carrie in the window. "Your turn," he said.

Carrie stuck her head out of the window. The corner of the house seemed to be a long way away.

"Try not to look down," Jon said. "I'll catch your legs."

She heard something from somewhere behind her. It was some movement on the stairs. Then a voice called, "Carrie? Jon? Are you up there?"

"They're coming!" she said.

She pushed herself out the window, then slid her legs around and down the wall so that she was dangling against the logs, hanging by her hands. Then she swung her legs toward the corner. Jon grabbed on to her knee, pulled her over next to him, and placed her feet on the crossed logs. "OK," he said. "Now let go of the sill and reach for my hand." She reached for his hand, and he grabbed on tight. Then she let go.

He pulled her upright. "You OK?" he asked.

"Yeah." She took a few deep breaths. "I'm OK. Now let's climb down and get the hell out of here."

Jon heard the bedroom door bang open against the wall and heard Chestnut enter the room. He looked over at Carrie and shook his head. "We're not going to make it."

# Chapter 32

Ana Chestnut stepped through the doorway, scanned the room, and saw the open window. Looking outside, she saw its screen lying on top of the roof to the porch. She gauged the distance to the corner of the house and its ladder of crossed logs, and she saw how they'd escaped. Then she called down to her partner, "Chap, they've fooled us. They've climbed out a window and down to the ground. Don't let them get to their car. They're going to try to get away."

Chestnut leaned farther out of the window. Jon and Carrie were nowhere in sight. Alvord pulled his gun and chambered a round. He burst out through the front door, gun in hand, extending the gun out in front of him. The car was still there. He ran to the passenger-side windows and looked inside. It was unoccupied. He tried the doors. They were locked. He scanned the clearing down to the tree line. They weren't there. Then he glanced back toward the house.

"Ana, can you hear me?"

Chestnut's voice came from the window at the back of the house. "I can hear you."

"They aren't here. Do you see them?"

"No, I don't, but they could be on the porch or pressed up against the house where my view is blocked by the roof. The route to the trees is clear."

He said, "They're around here somewhere. Their car's still here. I need some help."

"I'll be right down." She started to move.

"Clear the house first. They could've used the open window as a decoy."

Chestnut checked each of the bedrooms. She had her gun in her hand. She cleared the second floor and then moved down the stairs. She checked the rest of the house, found the door to the electronics room and the back door still locked, and then stepped outside. She approached Alvord and said, "They probably heard the car when we drove up. They must've seen us through the master bedroom window and then made their escape. If they'd been on the first floor, they'd have gone out through the back, and that door's locked. They must've unlocked the window, kicked out the screen, and climbed down where the notched logs come together."

Alvord moved his attention away from the clearing to the periphery of the house. "They can't have been gone long," he said. "I don't think there's been time enough for them to reach the trees. You stay here with the car. I'll check around back." Alvord started around the left side of the house. Chestnut turned her gun toward the right.

Alvord moved slowly and deliberately. His gun was extended in front of him. He carefully moved one step at a time in a shooter's crouch, scanning back and forth as he moved. In all probability his adversaries weren't armed, but he'd learned from years of experience to be careful.

He maintained his position at a distance of fifteen feet from the house as he moved, close enough for him to see both on and under the porch and far enough away so that neither Jon nor Carrie would have an opportunity to jump him from a hiding place. He disappeared around the corner. Chestnut stood her ground, blocking their way to the car from the other side.

The left side of the house was clear; so was the route to the tree line. Alvord quickly turned the corner and moved around to the back. He approached the back door, pulling the latch up with his left hand while holding the gun in his right. The door was locked and secure. The rest of the back of the house was clear.

There were several large stumps—large enough to hide behind—in the space between the back of the house and the tree line. Alvord called out, "Jon, Carrie, are you there?"

Nothing. There was no response.

He raised his gun and fired a shot into one of the stumps.

**BANG!**

Still nothing.

"Come out, come out, wherever you are."

There was no movement, no noise.

He watched for a moment more and then moved on.

He moved to the far corner leading to the remaining unchecked side of the house. He braced himself and then snapped his gun around in front of him as he pivoted to the right. They weren't there. He checked the remaining hiding places on the right side. Nothing. "Shit! Ana!" He sprinted to his left as he yelled.

"What?"

"Come back here. Hurry. They're behind one of these stumps." She ran around to join him. "The periphery of the house is clear, and there wasn't enough time for them to make the tree line, so they've got to be behind one of those stumps." They moved out into the clearing. "Cover me."

Chestnut took a central position while Alvord moved from stump to stump to stump. She kept her gun level. There were seventeen large stumps spread out between the house and the tree line. Alvord checked each of them in turn. When he finished, he rejoined Chestnut.

"Nothing?" she asked.

"Nothing. What about the outbuilding?"

"It was locked, but I'll check it again." Chestnut jogged around to the front and checked the outbuilding door. It was still locked. She circled the building and emerged from the other side just as Alvord joined her. "Nothing there, either," she said.

"Where the hell are they?"

They both gazed out toward the tree line. "I don't know how they did it, but they must've made it to the trees." She looked back at Alvord. "We blew it. We blew it big time. There's no finding them now."

Alvord scanned the trees as he answered, "I agree. As good as this place is, it's not perfect. Last year they built a cell tower down by the hatchery. We're within cell coverage." He moved over to Jon's Explorer, jimmied the hood open, did something to the ignition system, and then closed the hood again. "OK, there. They won't be driving in this for a while. Now, any bright ideas?"

"Our cover's blown, our subjects have escaped, and we've lost our opportunity. No doubt they've told someone they were coming up here. We aren't going to find them any time soon. We've made good money on this deal, and I think it's time to cash in. We ought to get the hell out of here before they have a chance to contact someone for help. We go to plan B."

Alvord took one last look around the clearing. Jon and Carrie were nowhere in sight. Then he and Chestnut climbed into the Ford and made their exit.

# Chapter 33

JON LET OUT his breath. He and Carrie looked down from the roof. They'd climbed up the corner of the house, not down, and now they watched as the government-issue car slowly disappeared beyond the tree line. "What's plan B?"

When they'd heard the bedroom door bang open against the wall, they'd quickly changed direction and climbed up to the roof. Its cedar shakes were slippery with years of accumulated moss, and they'd had a hard time pulling themselves up over the edge. They'd barely made it when Chestnut stuck her head out the window. They'd flattened themselves against the shingles and held their breath when she'd called down to her partner. She was only a few feet away. Fortunately for them, she didn't look up.

After she'd pulled her head back inside, they'd slithered up the slippery shingles to the peak of the roof, where they'd hoped to gain a better vantage point. Then they'd watched Alvord as he searched the perimeter of the house. They thought they'd been spotted when Chestnut searched around the outbuilding. She'd seemed to look right at them, but the sun was behind them, and either she'd missed them entirely or she hadn't registered what she'd seen because of the glare. Finally they'd watched as she and Alvord climbed into their car and drove away.

Jon crawled a little farther up on the peak of the roof to make sure that his adversaries were gone. He took a deep breath and then let it out again. They were nowhere in sight. He let his head fall back with a sigh. He rolled to his side and tried to relax his tense muscles.

"Do you think they've really left?" Carrie asked. She was still flattened low to the roofline.

"Yeah, I think so, at least for now." He rolled onto his back.

"Well, don't get too comfortable," she said. "We've got to figure out how to get off of this roof and out of here." She pushed herself up with the palms of her hands. "Do you have your cell phone?"

"It's in the car," he answered. He rolled back onto his stomach and scanned the area in front of the house. His eyes followed the path to where Alvord's car had disappeared into the trees. "Maybe I should go get it." He raised his head up a little farther and started to move.

"Let's wait just a minute." She held out her hand in front of him. "They did something to your car. And then there's the plan B thing. Maybe they did it to lure us out into the open. They might be waiting just beyond the trees trying to trap us."

Jon studied the tree line. He couldn't see any sign of the marshals. "I don't think so," he answered. Then he looked up at the sky. "The sun's going to go down soon. It's going to get cold." He looked back at the tree line. It looked quiet. "I'm going to climb down."

"Jon." She put her hand on his shoulder. "Let's wait."

He studied her for a moment and then nodded OK. Forty-five minutes later he started inching down the roof.

:　　:　　:

The roof was slippery, and Jon had to be careful. He climbed down the logs on the back left corner of the house to remain hidden from the road. Then he worked his way along the edge of the porch. His car was about thirty feet away from the corner of the house. He stopped at the corner to assess his situation, looked around, and whispered to himself, "So far, so good." Carrie watched his progress from the protection of her perch.

The space between the house and the car was exposed and open to view from the trees. He had no choice but to momentarily reveal his position, and if the marshals were in the trees, they would see him. He got ready to run. He took a deep breath and exhaled. Then he took another and then another. Finally he hunched down, launched himself toward his car, and closed the distance in a running half-crouch as fast as he could. He flattened himself against the side of the car away from the trees when he got there.

He remained still for a moment.

He caught his breath. Then he popped up to look through the car door window and across to the clearing through the window on the other side. There was no sign of either Alvord or his partner. He popped back down again.

He reached into his pocket for his keys and then unlocked the driver's-side door. He opened it just enough to slip inside. The cell phone was in one of the cup holders. He reached across, took it out, and flipped it open. His LCD indicated a good signal. He hit speed dial number one. Karen answered on the fourth ring. "Seattle Police Department, Detective Able speaking."

"Karen, listen, we're at the safe house."

"Jon, what's wrong?" She could hear the tension in his voice.

"The marshals, Alvord and the other one, aren't who they say they are. They're the impostors from Ocean City, and they're trying to kill us."

"What?"

"Carrie says Alvord is the guy who claimed to be Dr. Bennett, the one who conned her into killing Frankie Wolfson. The other one pretended to be Wolfson's wife. Carrie tagged them right away." Jon quickly described their situation. "You've got to help us, and fast. They did something to my car, and I don't think it'll start. I don't want to try it because I don't want to make the noise."

"The marshals are trying to kill you?"

"That's what I said."

"Jon, don't move. Just sit tight. I'll get someone out there as fast as I can."

He gave her the directions to the safe house. "And tell them not to fuck around, will you? We're kind of exposed here."

"I'll tell them. Hold on. Be careful." Karen broke the connection.

# Chapter 34

CARRIE WAS THE first to see the flashing lights approaching from her perch on the rooftop. There were three sets—three cars from the King County Sheriff's Department. First she heard the sirens, and then she saw the lights. The cars exploded out of the tree line and bounced and banged their way up the path toward the house. Deputy Pigott arrived first. He spun his lead car to the side and slid to a stop with his driver's-side door away from Jon's Explorer. Then he jumped out of the car with his pistol in his hand. He used his car as a shield, braced his arm on its top, and pointed his gun at Jon. The two other cars slid into position in rapid succession, bracketing the first. Jon carefully got out of his Explorer with his hands in the air.

"Jon Kirk?" Pigott asked.

"Yeah, that's me. I'm the one who called the police." Jon stood with his hands up. He moved out in front of his car. Pigott kept his gun trained on the center of his chest. "I'll just get my wallet out of my pocket and show you my ID."

"Do it slowly," Pigott instructed. "Don't make any sudden moves."

Jon slowly reached back to his hip pocket and very deliberately removed his wallet. Then he took his driver's license and press card out of the wallet and held them out in front of him. Deputy Pigott checked to make sure that the other deputies had Jon clearly in their sights, and then he came out from behind the protection of his car. He approached Jon and took the ID. After checking it he asked, "Where's the other one, Dr Williams? There were supposed to be two of you."

Without turning, Jon pointed up over his shoulder and behind him toward the peak of the roofline. Pigott looked up. Carrie shyly waved to him from the top of the roof.

"Carrie Williams?" Pigott asked.

Carrie nodded, and then she started to climb down the other side.

Pigott then asked, "Is everyone all right?"

Jon finally relaxed his arms and lowered them to his sides. "Yeah, we're OK. We were lucky. It could've turned out differently."

Pigott put his gun away. He wanted to know what was going on, why they were out there, and what this place was. The other deputies came out from behind their cars.

Jon told him the bare minimum. He wanted to save what he could for his newspaper story. If things worked out right, he'd have a major exclusive. The electronic media would break things first, of course. There was no way to stop that, but he'd have the details, and he didn't want some blabby cop ruining it all.

Carrie appeared from around the side of the house just as he'd started to talk. She had a big tear in her slacks along her left inseam. Jon could see blood running down from a wound near her knee. She followed his eyes down to the tear. "I caught it on a nail," she said. "It's nothing. It doesn't even hurt." She walked over to join Jon and the deputy.

"You're going to need a tetanus shot for that," Jon said.

"And you got your medical license when?" She smiled at Jon and then at Pigott.

"Deputy Pigott," Jon said by way of introduction, "this is Dr. Carrie Williams. She's the reason we're all here." He turned to Carrie. "Carrie, I was just explaining to Deputy Pigott how we came to be here." He then continued with his abridged version of their story. Fifteen minutes later Karen's car broke out from the tree line and tore into the clearing.

# Chapter 35

KAREN WAS BACK in her office at the Public Safety Building when Robbie Washington walked in and plopped himself down in a chair. He'd just finished his interviews with Jon and Carrie. He'd questioned them separately and had spent over an hour with each. Karen greeted him and then sat down on a corner of her desk. She dangled her legs over the edge, kicked off her shoes, and asked, "Learn anything?"

"No surprises," Robbie answered. "By the way, I think you did right by letting me do the interviews. You had too much of a conflict of interest. It got kind of crowded in there, anyway. We had both a deputy marshal from the Justice Department and the King County sheriff in attendance. Why they couldn't just sit on the other side of the mirror I'll never know." He brushed a piece of lint off the top of his left knee.

Karen crossed her ankles. "So what have we got?"

"Well, to start with, we've got a couple of dirty U.S. marshals." He picked away the last of the lint. "And secondly, we've got a pissed-off Justice Department.

"Marshal Carl Jensen confirmed that Alvord and Chestnut are the real deal, and after our interview with Carrie, he had to agree that they're the ones who impersonated Wolf's wife and Bennett. In all likelihood they're the ones who killed the records clerk in Ocean City, Candy Peterson, and Chester Dorsey as well. The feds are always surprised to find that their shit stinks just like everybody else's."

"We knew all of that four hours ago," Karen said. "We don't need to know what; we need to know why. Why would a U.S. federal marshal want to murder one of his own protected witnesses, especially one who was dying anyway?"

Robbie watched Karen rub the bottom of her foot. "Let's try this on for size," he finally answered. "Wolfson was a bookkeeper for the syndicate. He embezzled a bunch of their money. We know this to be a fact. He traded the Justice Department his promised testimony in court for a new identity, protection, and freedom from imprisonment. This also is a fact. The U.S. marshals that were assigned to protect him did their job and seemingly did it well until he became sick—fact three. Then the marshals turned, and as he neared death, they killed him, using Carrie Williams as a proxy."

"Uh-huh," Karen answered. "Fact four, but that doesn't get us any closer to why they did it. And as I said, we don't need what; we need why. We need a motive."

"I'm getting there. Just give me a minute. The only motive that makes sense, at least to me, is that they were trying to cover something up."

"Well, duh!" Karen again reached down to rub her foot.

Robbie continued, "Why do you kill an already-dying man?" He paused for effect, and then he answered his own question. "To shut him up." He raised his index finger in the air, indicating number one.

"Maybe," Karen said, "but it could've been something else, too, like revenge, but I'm with you so far. Go on."

"OK." Robbie shifted slightly forward. "Why, then, would they have needed to shut him up?" He raised a second finger. "Wolfson had something on them, something big, something they had to keep quiet at all costs." He looked into Karen's eyes and then widened his own. He wiggled his eyebrows.

She looked back at him blankly and shook her head.

He raised a third finger. "What is it that Wolfson did? Why did he need the protection of a new identity?" Robbie cocked his head to the side. "He embezzled one hundred million dollars. And who knew that he'd embezzled ..."

Karen interrupted. "They shook him down!" She hopped off the desk; then she started to pace. "They blackmailed him! They probably told him they'd blow his cover if he didn't pay. They'd let the syndicate know where he was."

"But then when he got sick?"

"They would've had to accelerate their plan. They would've wanted the rest of his money, all one hundred million of it." Karen paced over to the window, turned, and started back. Then she stopped still. She looked at Robbie. "They didn't have a choice, did they?" Robbie shook his head. "Frankie Wolfson never had a chance. At some point they had to decide to give up the money and kill him. There was no other way. It didn't matter whether they got the rest of the money or not. They couldn't risk his waking up and telling someone about the blackmail. They couldn't afford a sudden deathbed confession when he had nothing left to lose." She hopped back up on her desk. "And then when Carrie gave him a stimulant ..."

Robbie sat back in his chair. "It's not a bad theory."

"And it might even be right," Karen continued. "But what about the Grinstein syndicate? What about them?"

"What about them?" Robbie asked. "You seen any wise guys hanging around here lately?"

"Uh, I guess not," she answered. "OK, no wise guys, but what about Carrie?"

"Yeah, well, about Carrie, she was a loose end." He rubbed his chin and felt his five o'clock shadow. "Carrie could identify them, both Alvord and Chestnut. She picked them out of a photo line-up during her debriefing session. They couldn't have that. But they should've killed her earlier. It wouldn't have been that hard. There's something else going on here, something that made them want to keep her alive."

Karen said, "Maybe they saw something on the tapes."

"The tapes Jon stole from the hospital?"

"He says he didn't steal them; an anonymous informant gave them to him."

Robbie rolled his eyes. "Give me a break!"

"Anyway, the tapes clearly show Carrie giving Wolfson a stimulant and then turning off the sound. They would've wanted to know about the subsequent conversation, what Wolfson had said to her. Did he tell her about the blackmail, or maybe even about the money? What if he told her where she could find it? That would also explain Candy Peterson's torture and murder. She also spent a lot of time with Wolfson after he received his stimulant."

Karen tucked her hands under her thighs and started bouncing her legs. "Chestnut and Alvord trashed Carrie's apartment in Ocean City looking for something. Maybe it was something tied to the money. Whatever it was, they didn't find it. Otherwise they wouldn't still be after her."

"But maybe they did find it," Robbie answered. "They'd still have to shut her up. It's hard to know for sure. This thing's running in circles. Where's Carrie now?"

"They're on their way to my apartment. They'll be safe there, at least for the time being. I'm going to meet them there later. We'll keep them protected. Do you want me to call them?"

Robbie made a sniffing sound with his nose. "No, don't bother. It's just a theory, and it doesn't really matter anyway. She's not going to tell us anything more than she already has. We'll find out more when we catch our two itinerant marshals, and in all probability that won't take too long—not with the SPD, the state patrol, and the FBI all looking for them. They aren't going to get very far."

"I wouldn't be too sure about that," Karen said as she hopped off her desk. She smoothed the wrinkles from her skirt. "Hiding people was their business; remember? They're professionals, and they aren't going to make many mistakes. I'm not so sure they're going to be all that easy to find. It could take awhile."

Robbie stood up and shook his head. "This case gives me a headache." He moved toward the door.

"Robbie," Karen called out after him, "do you really think Carrie might know where Wolfson hid his money?"

# Chapter 36

"JON, I KNOW where the money is." It was Carrie.

Jon hit the brakes. "What?" He pulled over to the side of the road. One of the deputies had fixed his car while it was out at the safe house.

"I said I know where Wolfson hid his money. He told me about it in the hospital. He told me who he was and what he'd done."

Jon stared at her for a moment. "Goddamn!"

"Yeah, goddamn! So what do you say? We've been messing around long enough. Let's go get it."

Jon's mouth dropped open.

"I need your help. I can't get it by myself."

Jon was stunned. He stared at her for a moment more. He closed his mouth. "You know where Wolfson's money is?"

"That's what I said. What is it about that concept that you don't understand?"

Jon squinted and wrinkled his forehead. "What about the police?"

"Haven't told them yet. There's going to be a reward, potentially a big one, and I want to work that out before …"

"Carrie?"

"We're not going to *keep* the money. That'd be stupid. There's no problem there."

"Carrie, how'd you get Wolfson to tell you?"

"Look, it went like this. Wolfson was oversedated by his doctor, and as I told you, I gave him a stimulant so we could talk. We talked about his living will and about his wish to die. He was a little fuzzy about the living will, but he told me in no uncertain terms that he was ready to end his life. He'd felt humiliated by his disease, and he wanted it over with. We talked details. He wanted to know what medications I would use. He wanted to know what he would feel. I explained it all to him as best I could. Then he called me closer, and his voice dropped to a whisper. He knew about the audiovisual system but not that I'd already turned off the sound. He thanked me for taking care of him, and then said he had a favor to ask. That's when he told me about the money he'd stolen.

"I was totally surprised. I thought he was Stewart Wolf, a local retiree. I didn't know what to say. I just listened and let him talk.

"He told me that he didn't want the government to get the money, that it really wasn't theirs anyway, and that he didn't want the Grinstein syndicate to get it, either. I had no idea who they were back then. He said he wanted me to have it. He wanted me to have all of it and to do with it whatever I wanted. He told me I could keep it, spend it, give it to charity, whatever."

"Carrie."

"And then he told me where it was."

"Jesus, Carrie, do you know how much money we're talking about here? Wolfson hid almost one hundred million dollars."

"More, actually," she answered. "Quite a bit more. Tens of millions more."

Jon seemed nervous. He started to fidget. "And you want me to help you get it?"

"I can't do it by myself. If I could, I would."

He unconsciously started playing with the clasp on his seatbelt. He clicked it open and then reconnected it. "I don't know." He clicked it again.

"Jon, it's a hell of a story."

"I know." He clicked his clasp one more time and then took his hands off his seatbelt.

"It'd be your exclusive," Carrie continued.

"Uh-huh."

A FedEx truck zoomed by only a foot or so away from the side of their car.

Carrie waited a moment and then gave Jon a shove. "Come on, Jon. What do you say?"

"I said I don't know. I'm thinking." Several more cars passed by. "What about Wolfson's former employers? They'll want their money back. You don't want to mess around with those guys, do you?"

"I told you I don't plan on keeping it. Once we turn it in, there's nothing they can do. It'll be over. They're professionals. They won't bother me after that; there'd be no point."

Jon thought a moment more; then he said, "I'll have to call Karen."

"Go ahead; call her. Ask her for her permission. Invite her along if you want."

Jon's lip twitched. "I don't have to ask her for her permission!" He got out his cell phone and speed-dialed Karen's number.

"By the way, you didn't tell me where we're going." The phone connected and immediately switched into Karen's voice mail. She must have been talking to somebody else.

"You haven't agreed to help me yet."

Jon didn't leave a message; instead he broke the connection. He'd call her back later. "Let me make sure I understand this," he said. "The money goes back."

"That's right; the money goes back."

"There's a reward in it for you and a story for me. That's all; that's the deal."

"That's the deal."

"Nothing else?"

"Nothing else."

"You're sure?"

"I'm sure."

He took in a breath and then slowly let it out through his pursed lips. "OK, then I guess that's it. Count me in." He put his hands on the steering wheel. "Where are we going?"

"Uh, how about to the nearest gas station?" She nodded toward the gas gauge. The needle was pegged on empty, and the low-fuel red light was on.

Jon checked the low-fuel light. "Good idea." They pulled away from the curb and drove to the gas station on James St.

:   :   :

Jon got out and began fueling his car. Carrie sat inside and watched as the numbers ticked away on the pump. She'd done her research. Jon had a reputation; he was the reporter who'd do anything for a story. She could count on that, couldn't she? She needed his help. Wasn't that why she'd contacted him in the first place? She bit her lip, opened her window, and leaned outside. "Jon?"

"Just a minute." He finished fueling the car. "I need to clean the windshield. It's got bugs all over it." He wiped off the windshield and then climbed back inside. "OK, what?" He turned to face her.

"We have to go to Ocean City."

"No problem. We'll get there a little after dark. I'll call in and tell the paper I won't be in tomorrow. Anything else?"

"We're going to the Pacific Northwest Forensics Laboratory."

Jon raised an eyebrow. "The Pacific Northwest Forensics Laboratory? The place where the feds study decaying bodies?"

"That's the place."

"Mavis told me about that. They partially bury bodies and body parts there. They put them in varying soil conditions so they can study how they rot. They count the worms and stuff in the tissues at different time intervals after death so they can figure out how long discovered bodies have been dead. Alex Morse set it up. The hospital supplies the bodies."

"I didn't know that. Wolfson certainly knew what he was doing. Who'd want to go wandering around a place like that?"

Carrie checked the look on Jon's face. "This isn't going to be a problem, is it—the decaying corpses, I mean?

The woman at the pump ahead of them started her engine. She checked her rearview mirror and drove away.

"Decaying corpses? Of course not!" Jon turned the key in the ignition. "Why would it bother me? They're just dead bodies." He pulled out of the gas station and drove toward the interstate.

# Chapter 37

THE DRIVE TO Ocean City took about four-and-a-half hours. Jon had tried to call Karen several times during their drive, but he hadn't been able to connect. He'd get a dial tone on his cell phone, and the signal strength display indicated that he was well within range of a cell tower, but the calls wouldn't go through. There was something wrong with his service. After a stop in Centralia for some food, he called Karen on a landline, but she wasn't available. They drove on toward their destination in Ocean City.

"Where to now?" Jon asked after they crossed into the Ocean City city limits. The sun had long since set, and the sky was dark and overcast. His headlights cut a path through a light layer of ground fog.

"Follow the highway all the way out to the bridge and then turn left. We're going to take the coast highway south. The laboratory should be a short distance up an unmarked asphalt road somewhere near the seventeen-mile mark."

It took Jon three tries to find the right road. After approximately a quarter of a mile, they came to a ten-foot-tall gate and chain link fence. The fence extended out of sight into the darkness in both directions. Its gate was locked with a large steel padlock, and both the fence and the gate were topped with coiled razor wire. A sign on the gate read:

## PACIFIC NORTHWEST FORENSICS LABORATORY
## FEDERAL BUREAU OF INVESTIGATION
## UNITED STATES DEPARTMENT OF JUSTICE
## AUTHORIZED PERSONNEL ONLY

Jon stopped the car and stared at the sign. He felt a cold shiver traverse the length of his spine. "You're sure the money's in there?" he asked. He wasn't OK with the thought of decaying bodies, even in the name of forensic science.

"I never told you the money's in there," Carrie answered. "We're looking for a key, the key to a safe deposit box."

"But it leads to the money?" Jon continued. "I'm not going in there unless we're going after the money."

Carrie rolled her eyes. "Yes, Jon," she answered, "we're going after the money. The key leads to the money. Now come on. Let's get this over with."

"OK, I just wanted to be sure." He looked back toward the fence. "That razor wire's going to be a problem. We're going to have to find something to throw over the top to protect us. There's no way we're going to be able to break that padlock." He focused on the wire coils. "Climbing the fence is our only way in."

Jon turned his headlights off. They were suddenly swallowed by an almost total absence of light. He reached across to the glove compartment, took out a flashlight, and turned it on. Carrie opened her door to get out; the interior lights made it seem even darker outside. Jon also got out, pulling his driver's-side floor mat out with him. He sized it up, comparing it to the coils of wire on the top of the fence. It was thick enough, but it clearly wasn't large enough. He reached up under the dashboard and started peeling the floor carpet away from its steel foundation.

"What are you doing?"

"Just watch."

It took him several minutes to get it separated and all the way out. Then he brought it over to the fence. There was more than enough carpeting to do the job. "Here," he said, handing it to Carrie. "Pass it on up to me when I get up there." He started to climb the links of the fence.

Jon climbed to a height where he could reach over the razor wire. Carrie climbed up three feet or so and passed him the carpet. Jon laid the carpet over the wire. He tested it to make sure that it was thick enough to protect him, and then he rolled over the carpet and onto the other side of the fence. "Be careful," he said. Carrie followed him up and over. Once they were both safely on the other side, he asked, "Where to from here?"

Carrie looked around. There was nothing but blackness outside the flashlight beam. "We need to find a small granite monument. It's supposed to look something like a headstone. It's the only one on the property. We're looking for a tin box just under the surface. It should be just behind the monument. The key's inside the box."

"A tin box under a headstone inside a cemetery? Haven't I seen this movie?" Jon felt another shiver. "I don't like this place."

"Oh, come on, Jon. There's nothing in here that can hurt you, at least not anymore."

"Uh-huh."

:   :   :

They followed the road on the other side of the gate through relatively open countryside to what looked like a World War II-style Quonset hut. The land was rocky, and stands of wind-stunted pine trees were scattered along the way. The trees were bent away from the ocean. There was a sliding door on the end of the building. It was unlocked, so Jon slid the door open. He illuminated the interior with his flashlight and then found a light switch. He switched it on.

The building was obviously a tool shed. Digging tools were located along one wall, and there were saws, large shears, other cutting tools, and an ax along another. There was a small tractor parked at the far end, and what looked like an old badly stained butcher block was in the middle. The plywood floor below the butcher block was also badly stained. "Are those stains blood?" Jon asked. His voice cracked a little.

Carrie ignored him. She checked the place out. Then she said, "There's nothing in here. Let's move on. We're wasting time." Jon shut off the light, and they moved back outside.

Jon searched the darkness with his flashlight. There were no trails or other marked paths to follow, so they set up a grid search pattern to look for the monument. Ground fog and rough terrain made the going slow. Their narrow flashlight beam scanned the ground in front of them, but it was diffused into the fog at distances greater than thirty feet.

After five minutes of searching, they caught a metallic reflection. It was the first man-made object they'd seen since the Quonset hit. As they approached it, they saw several others.

They were metal stakes that had been pounded into the

ground at irregular intervals. Each stake had a flat eight-by-ten-inch shiny metal plaque attached to its top.

Jon shone his flashlight on the plaques. Each one identified a body part such as an arm, head, or torso, along with a date and time of death and a date, time, and depth of burial. As they proceeded, they found other stakes with other identifications in other soil conditions.

Jon was having difficulty keeping his bearings in the fog. The air near the stakes felt heavy, with a faint smell of putrefaction. One of the plaques read, "Surface". Jon slid his flashlight beam toward the base of the stake. Something yellowish protruded up through the ground. Carrie moved some leaves away with her foot.

"What *is* that?" Jon asked.

She tapped the object with the side of her shoe. It squished. "Do you really want to know?"

Jon flashed the light back onto the plaque. It read, "Left foot and lower leg." He swallowed the rising bile in the back of his throat and quickly turned his light away.

Another fifteen minutes went by before they finally found the stone monument. It was located in front of a stand of seven wind-sculpted pines. About four feet high, it was made out of granite and rounded at the top like a tombstone, and it was set on a flat granite slab. A flowery epitaph on the front thanked the donors for their contributions to forensic science. "This is it," Carrie said. She immediately went around to the back.

The ground behind the stone was firm and was strewn with pebbles and small rocks. She brushed away the rocks with her fingers, but the ground was too hard to dig without some kind of a tool.

Jon knelt down beside her. He retrieved his pocketknife from his pocket and opened the blade. He started to pry the dirt away, and after only a few minutes he heard the scraping sound of metal on metal. Uncovering a metal lunchbox less than six inches under the surface, he dug the dirt away from its sides and unearthed his find. He shook it in his hands. A metallic object rattled inside. He handed it to Carrie. Carrie opened the box, and Jon aimed his flashlight.

The key lay in a corner. It was about two inches long and had an identification number engraved into its base.

Neither one of them said anything for a moment. Jon stared at the key. "Is this it?" He reached into the box and picked it up. He held it in his hand. The engraved identification number read, "MQ67C27315Z." "It seems somehow anticlimactic." He moved the light from the key up to Carrie.

Carrie's face was crinkled in a broad smile. "It fits a lock not more than ten miles away from here," she said. "Assuming I can work out the reward, I'm going to be rich, and you just scored the story of the year."

"Well, then," Jon said, tossing the key up in the air and then catching it again, "what are we waiting for? Let's get on with it. We've got a treasure to find." He pointed the flashlight toward the ground and started moving away from the monument. Carrie stood where she was. Jon shone the flashlight back in her direction when he saw that she wasn't coming with him.

Carrie discarded the lunchbox on the ground and then held out her hand, palm up. She wiggled her fingers in a beckoning motion.

"Oh, sure, how silly of me." Jon walked back and gave her the key. She put it into her pocket.

"Now we can get on with it," she said. They started back toward the shed on their way to the car.

# Chapter 38

CARRIE EXPLAINED HER plan as they drove up the highway. The key they'd found was for a safe deposit box at the Bank of America near the dock in Ocean City. Wolfson had rented it under the alias Terry Ring.

Jon would have to assume Ring's identity, walk into the bank with Carrie, ask to see his safe deposit box, and present his key. Then he'd have to sign a signature card, and his signature would be compared to the one that Wolfson had signed. He'd have to copy Wolfson's handwriting from the card while he signed Ring's name. It was imperative that the two signatures match well enough to fool the bank teller. Finally he'd have to tell them his personal password; it was supposed to be his mother's maiden name. Carrie would tell him the password when they got there. And then if everything went absolutely as planned, they'd leave the bank with somewhere in excess of one hundred million dollars' worth of Lichtenstein bearer stock certificates.

"Are you crazy?" asked Jon. "That's never going to work. They'd know right away that I'm not Wolfson. I don't look anything like him. We're not even close to the same age. What if they require a photo ID?"

"Oh, I don't think you'll have a problem." Carrie answered. "I doubt if Wolfson's been to the bank more than a handful of times over the past several years. He was banking under an alias, and he wouldn't have wanted to be recognized for who he really was. They won't remember what he looked like. And as for the signature, you should be able to passably copy it if you just take your time and don't get nervous."

"And the photo ID?"

"We can't worry about that. If they ask, they ask. Tell them you forgot your driver's license. They use signature cards to keep a signed record of who goes in and out of the vault. A valid signature might be enough; it depends on the teller. If they insist on a photo ID, just walk out."

"Just walk out?"

"Believe me, Jon, this is the only way. We're going to have to find a safe place to spend the night, and then we'll do it tomorrow."

"No." Jon shook his head. "We aren't doing this, not this way. Not only is it not legal; we'll get caught." The lights of Ocean City were visible ahead of them in the distance.

"We won't get caught!" Carrie's voice was emphatic. "What's the matter with you? This'll be the story of your career. And we both want to see what a hundred forty-five million dollars looks like."

Jon glanced across at her. "A hundred forty-five million?"

"That's right. A hundred forty-five million dollars and change."

Jon whistled through his teeth. "A hundred forty-five million!" He shifted his attention back to the road. "I should call Karen."

:   :   :

The fog was blowing in. Headlights from oncoming cars created a whiteout effect that made driving difficult. Jon reduced his speed further and drove on until he saw the glow from a neon sign. The sign read, "Ocean View Motel." A lighted *Vacancy* sign hung over the manager's office. There were only a few cars in the parking lot, and he'd already started to turn in to the driveway when he asked Carrie if this place was OK. She answered that it was. He rented a room for the night, then reparked his car near their unit. They were staying in number six. It was his lucky number.

Carrie took the key and opened the door. The place was small and clean, and it had two double beds. A TV with a cardboard sign on top advertised several pay-per-view channels. The clock radio by the bed came with a set of instructions so that guests could set their own alarms rather than order wake-up calls. The fog obscured the ocean view out of the back window.

Jon tried once again to reach Karen. This time he connected. "You're where with Carrie Williams?"

"In a motel room near Ocean City." He immediately pulled the phone away from his ear. Carrie could hear Karen's voice from half a room away. She was pissed! She was more than pissed. She was incredulous. She couldn't believe he'd gone after the money with Carrie on his own.

"We didn't get the money; we only found a key." He winced as he again pulled the receiver away from his ear. "No, we didn't call the police. We called you." Then he told her about the Pacific Northwest Forensics Laboratory and the safe deposit box key.

"You say the key goes to a safe deposit box at the local Bank of America?" Karen repeated.

"That's what Carrie says. The bank opens tomorrow at 10:00."

"OK. Jon. Listen, sit tight." She finally started to calm down. "I'll fly down early tomorrow. In the meantime, don't do anything. Do you understand? Those marshals may be still looking for you." Jon answered that he understood. "I'll contact Sergeant Tindall just as soon as we hang up. He'll get a court order for the bank to open the safe deposit box in the morning. He's bound to know a friendly judge. Tell Carrie she'll need to give me the key."

Jon put his hand over the receiver. "Karen says she can get a court order to open the box. She wants you to give her the key in the morning."

Carrie stared at him for a moment and then defiantly and emphatically shook her head. "No way! There's no way I'm giving her the key." She shook her head again. "She's not getting the key unless I can be there when they open the box. I've been through too much not to be there."

Jon took his hand away from the phone. "Karen, hold on a minute." Then he covered it again.

"Listen," Carrie continued. "This money is important to me. I'm setting up a fund in my mother's name. And I want to take care of Chester's family—Candy's, too. They need help and I feel responsible. I need to be there when they open it so they don't cheat me. The feds have done it before; I've checked. I want to be the one to personally turn it over to the police. That's not too much to ask, is it? I owe my mother that." When Jon didn't immediately answer, she repeated, "Is it?"

Jon uncovered the receiver again. "Karen, it's this way." He told her Carrie's condition. When she answered that she could work with it, he added, "And Carrie wants me to be there, too. That's another condition." Carrie gave him a quizzical look.

"Sure, why not?" Karen answered. "Let's have a party. I can't wait to hear what Sergeant Tindall has to say about this.

"And by the way, while you've been away playing around in graveyards, things have really been popping around here. The FBI accountants have uncovered two $50,000 wire transfers into Marshal Alvord's bank account; one dates from January and the other one from June. They're both from offshore numbered accounts. They're working on a trace. In any case, that's way more money than could possibly be accounted for from his government salary. It looks like he was working Wolfson with a classic shakedown. They're currently checking Chestnut's records, and I'd be surprised if they didn't find the same thing there. I'll bring copies of the documentation along when I come down, just in case we need it with our judge. I'll plan to get there around 7:00. With any luck we'll get the warrant and get to the bank before it opens at 10:00. Now what's the name Wolfson used for the account?"

Jon paused a moment and then answered, "Ring. Terry Ring."

"Where have I heard that name before? There's something fishy about that name."

"Fishy?"

Karen then said that she'd meet them the next morning, along with Tindall, in front of the bank at 10:00.

# Chapter 39

Jon and Carrie drove to the bank. They parked directly across the street from the front entrance. The street was busy with people. Neither Karen nor Tindall was anywhere in sight. Jon checked his watch; it was 9:45.

"Do you see them anywhere?" Carrie asked. "I don't see them. They should be here by now."

"I don't see them, either." Jon checked the street. He looked first to his left and then to his right. "They're not here."

"Maybe they had trouble with the judge."

"I wouldn't think so," Jon said. "The warrant request seems straightforward enough to me. They'll show. They're just a little late; that's all." He checked his watch again. It was 9:46.

A young woman in a red dress stepped out of a bookstore and into the flow of pedestrian traffic. A funny-looking old man who looked to be in his sixties walked his bearded collie along the docks. His pants were a little high-water. A garbage truck rumbled by. A short line formed near the door to the bank. It was 9:51.

Carrie said, "I still don't see them. Something's happened."

"Relax, Carrie. Nothing's happened. They're just a little late, that's all." He again scanned the street. "They'll be here."

A woman unlocked the door to the bank from the inside. The group of people waiting out front streamed in. A man in a suit stepped outside, looked around, and then went back inside. Jon checked his watch. He looked over at Carrie. "They opened early," he said.

"Maybe your watch is slow," she answered. She checked her own watch. It read 10:03. There was still no sign of either Karen or Tindall. "Maybe we should go to plan B."

"And that is?"

"I don't know. I'm working on it."

"I'm going to call Karen." He dialed her cell phone. It rang four times.

No answer.

Another five minutes passed; then an Ocean City police car pulled up in front of the bank. Tindall got out. He was eating a doughnut. He looked around. Jon spotted him right away. "Is that Sergeant Tindall?" Carrie asked.

"Has to be."

"Where's Karen?"

"I don't know; let's find out." They opened their car doors, got out, and crossed the street. Tindall saw them approach and quickly finished his doughnut. Jon asked him about Karen.

Tindall swallowed. "I left her at the courthouse. She was trying to get the judge to release some medical records. She'll be along pretty soon." He wiped off the corner of his mouth and then turned to Carrie. "So you're Carrie Williams." He looked her over. "The last time we talked, I asked you to keep me apprised of your whereabouts. It was a simple request; what happened?"

"Sorry," Carrie said. "Someone tried to kill me, and I got kind of busy. They got two of my friends." Her tone was indignant. A blue van sped by.

"All the more reason for you to have come in." Tindall eyed the van and judged it to be going about fifteen miles per hour over the speed limit. "You still owe me an interview. How about we do it after we finish here? Today!"

Jon interrupted, "Carrie, you don't have to ..."

She held up her hand. "Jon, it's OK. I don't mind, really. As a matter of fact I want to do the interview. I want to get it over with. I hate having things hanging over my head, and in any case I have nothing to hide."

"Very well," Tindall said. "Then that's it. We'll go to my office as soon as we're finished here. And now that that's settled," he said as he watched the speeding van turn the corner, "let's go into the bank and see what Frankie Wolfson has in his safe deposit box. Karen said you'd both be coming along."

"Shouldn't we wait for her?" Jon asked.

"I don't really see any need. You do have the key, don't you?" Carrie indicated that they did. "Good. Karen should be along any minute now, and she can join us inside when she gets here. I have the search warrant." He patted his breast pocket. "The bank knows we're coming. They know what they have to do."

"Then let's get on with it," Carrie said. Jon hesitantly agreed. He scanned the street in both directions, looking for Karen as they walked into the bank.

Carrie opened the door and went in first. Tindall followed closely behind. Jon waited a moment and then brought up the rear. Several people were lined up at the teller stations. There were surveillance cameras all over the place. Jon could see nine of them, and there were probably more. One of the cameras was directed toward the main entrance, one toward the entrance to a side office with an INVESTMENT SERVICES sign on the door, and another four toward the four teller stations. A thick, probably bulletproof, floor-to-ceiling plastic partition enclosed the teller stations, along with a supporting space in the back. A keypad-encoded secure door opened into the enclosed space, and a single camera watched both the keypad lock and the door. Two more cameras were located in the corners of the far wall on either side of the safe deposit vault. The bank manager's office was next to Investment Services.

The bank manager's door was open, and she was sitting at her desk. Tindall approached with his search warrant.

"I've been expecting you," she said. She inspected the warrant. "This is my copy to keep?" She put the warrant down on her desk.

"It's yours," Tindall answered. She slid it into the desk.

"You brought the key?"

"Here." Carrie reached into her purse, fumbled around a moment, retrieved the key, and then handed it to her.

"Good, follow me." She led them out of her office and over to the open safe deposit vault.

The massive vault door was made out of what looked to be polished stainless steel. You could see its locking mechanism through heavy glass panels on the back. An inner gate made out of vertical metal bars led to the interior of the vault, and it was closed. It locked with a simple lock. The manager unlocked the lock, and they went inside. "The area over there to the right is where we usually sign people in," she said. "No need for that this morning. We'll go all the way inside."

Hundreds of stainless-steel hinged safe deposit doors lined the sides and the back of the bank vault; the individual locked doors were of varying sizes. Each safe deposit door had two keyholes, one for the bank's key and one for the owner's key. Both keys were needed to open the doors. The bank manager moved over to the one numbered 87. It was one of the smallest ones. She inserted both keys in the door and turned them both to the right. Then she removed a long narrow box. "Here you are." She handed the box to Sergeant Tindall. Then she gave the owner's key back to Carrie. "I'm required by bank policy to observe as you open the box and inspect its contents. Why don't you follow me over to one of our private rooms?" She led the way.

She led them to a private room just around the corner to the right, and once they were all inside, she closed the door. "Lock it," Carrie said. She locked the door. Tindall put the box down on the table.

Jon eyed the box sitting in front of him. "Kind of small, isn't it?"

"Just open it." Carrie reached for the box.

"I'll do that," Tindall said. He blocked Carrie's arm and opened the box. He flipped back the lid. He searched its interior. He looked at the others in the room. "There's nothing in here!"

The lid to the box was hinged at the halfway point across its top, and Tindall folded it all the way back on itself. He shook the box. Nothing fell out. He stuck his hand inside, feeling into its back corners. It was empty. He turned it over and then turned it right side up again. He shook his head.

"Excuse me." The bank manager removed a small flashlight from a pocket in her skirt. "May I?" She shone the light into the box. It was indeed empty.

"Give me that!" Carrie grabbed it away. She shook it hard and explored its interior. Then she slammed it down on the desk. "We came all of this way!" She pushed it away. "Damn it, Frankie! People died for what was supposed to be in there!"

"Maybe it's something with the box itself," Jon said. "There has to be a message here somewhere." He picked up the box and turned it over in his hands. He paid attention to its surfaces. He inspected every side. He tilted it so that the light shone inside to the back.

"What about the hinge?" Carrie said. "Maybe there's something in the hinge."

"It would help if I knew what we were looking for," Tindall said. "I thought we were supposed to find a stack of bearer stock certificates."

"Look for a number," Carrie said. "Maybe there's a number. It could be on something that's rolled up and stuffed in the hinge. Maybe it's on microfilm or a microdot."

Jon checked the hinge. He tried to pull out its pin. It was solid; it wouldn't budge. There was nothing there.

He put the box back down on the table. "Well," he said to the empty box, "I have to hand it to you, Frankie." He started to chuckle. "It looks like the joke's on us."

"I don't see what's so damn funny!" Carrie said. "Candy and Chester are dead." She tilted the box up to look inside one last time and then shoved it back down onto the table. "I just can't believe that Frankie, or Stewart, or whatever his name was could lie to me on his deathbed. This just isn't right!"

"Settle down," Tindall said. "There's no need to raise your voice." The bank manager nodded.

Carrie snorted, then said to Jon, "Give me your car keys. I've got to get out of here. I've had enough of this claustrophobic room. I'll meet you in the car." She stood up. Jon gave her his keys.

"Maybe I should come with you," Tindall said. "I wouldn't want you to forget about our interview." He stood with her.

"Suit yourself."

Jon again picked up the box. Carrie unlocked the door, and she and Tindall left the room.

"Are we finished here?" the bank manager asked.

"Just a few more minutes," Jon answered. After he finished his final inspection, he said, "Here," and handed the metal box back to the bank manager. "Thank you for your help."

She answered, "You're very welcome." Then Jon left the room.

He walked out the front door, and as he left the bank, he noticed that Tindall's police car was still parked out front. Carrie was sitting in his Explorer across the street. He walked over to his car and opened the door. "Man, can you believe that?" he said to her. He climbed in behind the wheel. He started to say something else when he felt a sharp stabbing pain on the top of his right shoulder. He instinctively looked around. Someone's hand was holding a hypodermic syringe. A thumb was pressing on its plunger. Its needle was sticking through his clothes into his shoulder. That seemed strange.

He heard a voice from somewhere behind him say, "Do you think he's out yet?"

Another voice, a woman's voice, said, "Give him a few more seconds and then pull him into the back seat. It's time to quit fucking around."

He felt two arms from the back grasp him around the chest. Then nothing.

# Chapter 40

Jon woke up in a chair. His head hurt like hell. It throbbed in time with his heartbeat. He tried to reach up to rub his temple, but his arm wouldn't move; it was taped to the arm of his chair. He'd been tied to a wooden armchair with duct tape. His forearms had been taped to the arms, his calves had been taped to the legs, and several loops of tape had bound his waist to its back. Carrie was bound in a similar fashion to a chair about five feet to his right. She was still unconscious. They were sitting in the middle of what looked to be the living room of a small house.

"Carrie?" His voice was croaky and his mouth was dry. He cleared his throat and tried it again. "Carrie?" She didn't move. Her head was down on her chest. Her mouth was open. "Carrie, can you hear me?"

They were facing the front door. The room was painted a creamy white and was furnished with modest functional furniture. The curtains were drawn.

Jon pulled against his restraints. They held tight. He rocked in his chair. It moved. He scooted it a little closer to Carrie. "Carrie, wake up." He spoke in a half-whisper. There was no response.

Jon again started to work against the duct tape. He moved his arms from side to side and then pulled against the tape with his legs. He leaned forward, pushing down with his toes and lifting the front legs of his chair off the ground. The tape around his ankles seemed to stretch a little. He tried it again, wiggling from side to side at the same time. It felt to him that the tape loosened a little more. He rocked back on his heels, twisted his arms and body, and then went up on his toes again. The momentum carried him forward. Then he jerked to his right. The chair went over with a loud bump. He was lying on his side, still taped to the chair about three feet away from Carrie, when he heard footsteps approaching him from behind.

"My, my, aren't you the feisty one?" It was a female voice. She pulled him upright. She was strong. Then she pushed him into his original position about five feet away from Carrie.

Jon strained to see her. "Where are we?"

Ana Chestnut stood behind him with her hands on the back of his chair. "Now what could that bit of information possibly matter to you?" She noticed Jon glance over at Carrie, who was still unconscious. "Don't worry about her," Chestnut said. "She'll wake up in a few minutes. She'll be fine."

Jon tried to clear his throat. "What do you want from us?"

"Oh, come on now, Jon, really!" Chestnut let go of Jon's chair and moved over to Carrie. She stood in front of her, bent slightly at the waist. She was very close.

"Carrie?" Her voice was quiet. There was no response. She shook her head. "It seems like it's always this way," she said to Jon. Then she sighed, pulled Carrie's head up off her chest by her hair, and gazed into her glazed eyes for a moment. Then with a quick, sharp motion, she viciously smashed the heel of her hand into the left side of Carrie's face just in front of her left ear. It was a blow designed to cause maximal pain. Carrie's head snapped to the side; her body jerked; her eyelids fluttered. Chestnut did it again, but Carrie wouldn't wake up.

"These black ones," Chestnut said as if explaining things to Jon. "Sometimes it takes a lot to bring them around. I don't think their nerve endings are as sensitive as ours." She hit her a third time and then looked into her lolling eyes. When Chestnut saw no further response, she flung Carrie's head back down onto her chest. "This may take a little longer than I thought." She walked over to face Jon. "Your turn?" His eyes widened. She studied him for a moment, and then without saying anything further, she walked out of the room.

Jon resumed his struggle against his restraints. The tape on his arms held tight, but he made a little progress with the tape on his legs. He was able to turn his right ankle from side to side and to slide his leg up and down inside the tape. His waist was still firmly bound to the back of the chair.

Carrie started to move. She blinked her eyes and pulled her hand up against the tape restraints. She made a guttural sound.

"Carrie?" Jon said. She slowly turned her head to look at him. "Carrie, can you hear me?" She nodded her head. She tried to speak, but nothing came out. "Carrie, we've been drugged." He paused for her to take it in. "You're taped to a chair."

She stared at him for a moment, and then she looked down at her taped arms. She cleared her throat. She tried to say something, but her voice just croaked. The left side of her face hurt like hell. She swallowed and then swallowed again. She recognized the coppery taste of blood in her mouth. "How long have we been out?" she finally managed to ask. She had an unimaginable headache.

Jon answered, "I don't know."

A muffled voice from behind them said, "Chap, she's awake." It came from another room. Then two sets of footsteps approached.

:   :   :

Chap Alvord walked into the room; he carried a chair with him. He placed it directly front of Jon and Carrie, about six feet away. He assessed his captives. "Surprised?" he asked. "Come on, Jon. Don't tell me you're surprised to see us. You're smarter than that. Surely you know we've been on your trail the whole time. Plan B, remember? We tagged your car up at the safe house with a GPS beacon." He switched his gaze to Carrie. "And you—you at least should know better." Neither one of them answered. "You of course know why you're here." He turned his chair around backwards and sat down facing them. "Let's make this as simple as possible so that we can get this over with and all go home."

His voice became more forceful. "Where's the money?" Jon and Carrie looked at each other. Alvord paused a moment waiting for an answer. Neither one of them spoke. He persisted. "Tell me where the money is, and we'll forget that all of this unpleasantness ever happened."

"There is no money," Jon finally answered. "The safe deposit box was empty." Chestnut moved quickly in behind him and with a blur of motion struck a sharp blow to the side of his head. His head snapped to the side. It hurt like hell. He started to say something else when another blow caught him flush on his ear, knocking him and his chair over onto the floor. Chestnut pulled him up and then roughly pushed him back in place. He heard a loud ringing sound somewhere inside his head. He felt blood trickle down his neck from somewhere.

"I told you they'd say something like that," Chestnut said. She was still standing behind him.

"But it's true," Carrie insisted. "The box *was* empty."

"It's the truth," Jon echoed. Chestnut knocked him back down onto the floor. He braced himself for another blow when Alvord held up his hand, palm out, indicating that Chestnut should stop. She sat Jon back up and then slowly moved around to join Alvord.

"This isn't getting us anywhere," Alvord said, "and it's wasting time. Now, about the money ..."

"But," Carrie started to say.

Chestnut cut her off. "Shut the fuck up!"

Alvord glanced at Chestnut and then continued, "As I was saying, about the money. I want to explain to you exactly what's going to happen here. Here's what we're going to do." He leaned forward a little over the back of his chair. "I'm going to ask you a question, and then I'm going to allow a little time for you to consider your answer." He paused for effect. "And then, while you're thinking about your answer, Ana here is going to help you focus your thoughts." He paused again. "Ana's good at that. She's going to hurt someone, and not just a little bit, either—not like that little tap on the side of the face." His eyes flashed toward Jon. "She's going to hurt someone bad. She's going to cause someone to feel burning, intense pain. It's going to be the kind of pain that really focuses the mind." Chestnut was looking directly at Carrie. "And then, assuming we don't get the answer we're looking for the first time, she'll do it again, and again, and then again. It'll go on like that until you tell us exactly what we want to know."

Alvord sat back in his chair. "So is everyone ready?" Chestnut took her cue and started out of the room.

"This is insane," Jon protested. "We don't know anything!" A small bead of sweat formed on his temple. Carrie let out an involuntary whimper. Alvord answered with silence.

Chestnut returned a minute or so later with a large wrench and a foot-long section of heavy twine. She handed the twine and the wrench to Alvord. Then she left the room again.

"What are you going to do to us?" It was Carrie.

"To you?" A heavy scraping noise sounded from the room behind them and then moved in their direction. It was the sound of something being dragged across the hardwood floor. "Oh, no, not to you."

Chestnut appeared in Jon's peripheral vision and moved to his side. Alvord stood up. He walked over to Carrie. Alvord and Chestnut turned Carrie and Jon around 180 degrees at the same time.

There was Karen. She was shaking violently, nodding her head back and forth from side to side. She was facing them, duct-taped to a chair, arms to chair arms, legs to chair legs, and torso to the chair back. She tried to say something, but duct tape covered her mouth. She looked into Jon's eyes. Alvord walked over to Karen, stood beside her, and stilled her head. He pulled it over against the side of his chest and slowly ran his fingers through her hair. Then he said, "This is going to be ugly."

Jon shouted, "No! Don't do this!" He pulled against the tape holding him down.

Chestnut quickly moved close to Karen's left hand. Alvord moved away. Karen started to thrash against her restraints.

"Oh, hold still," Alvord said with a disgusted tone in his voice.

Then he turned to Jon. "We found her over by the courthouse. I think she was on her way to see you. She knows exactly what's going to happen to her."

Chestnut grabbed her hand and whipped the twine around her little finger, pulling it tight against the solid wooden arm of the chair. Alvord smiled. Karen looked away. Her eyes welled up with tears.

"The most sensitive nerve endings in the body are those farthest away from the central nervous system," Alvord said. "That's a fact. The periosteal nerves surrounding the small bones of the hand are the most sensitive of all. We agree with the Chinese on that point. They had that thing that they did with the fingernails." His eyes bored in on Jon. "Ana here is going to exploit that sensitivity," he continued. "Allow me to explain it to you.

"First she's going to crush the bones in Detective Able's little finger with this wrench." He pointed the wrench at Jon and then handed it to Chestnut. "And then once that's done, she'll work the shattered bone fragments around into the nerves. By that time, of course, Detective Able will be screaming. She'll scream uncontrollably. She'll scream like nothing you've ever heard before. She'll scream until she passes out. And then when she comes to, assuming you haven't given us the answers we want to hear, we'll do it again." He smiled. "All you'll need to do to stop it is to tell us what we want to know." Then he hardened his gaze. "So, now, tell us, where's the money?"

Jon pleaded with him. "We don't know anything about the money. We don't know where it is. The box was empty! Maybe there isn't any money." He turned to Carrie. "Carrie, tell them." He heard Karen whimper through the duct tape. He searched her face, her expression. She'd fixed her eyes on his. He cried out,

"For God's sake, stop this!"

Chestnut tightened her grip on the wrench. Jon thrashed in his chair. She lifted the wrench up above Karen's finger. Karen started to sob; she closed her eyes. Jon cried, "You bastards!" Chestnut brought the wrench down with a sickening whack. An anguished scream escaped through the duct tape covering Karen's mouth. Jon banged his chair back and forth. Chestnut pushed the handle of the wrench down on the shattered finger. She worked it from side to side, crunching the bone fragments into the nerves. Jon cried out. He twisted back and forth. He struggled against the tape. He banged his chair around on the hardwood floor. The screaming continued. It got louder. The duct tape could hardly hold it back. Then it stopped.

# Chapter 41

CHESTNUT PULLED THE twine from around Karen's mangled finger. It was swollen and disfigured. Her head hung to the side. Her eyes were partially open but were unfocused and glazed. Her hair was damp. Alvord walked over and put two fingers on the side of her neck. She didn't respond to his touch, but her pulse was strong. He glanced over at Chestnut. "You're scary, you know that?" He pulled his hand away. "Next time she'll start screaming as soon as she sees the wrench."

"Goddamn you!" Jon blubbered. Tears streaked down his face. "Look at her! Karen had nothing to do with this. She didn't do a damn thing, and look what you bastards did to her." Karen was limp in the chair. Her face was pale, her breathing barely perceptible.

"Oh, put a sock in it!" Alvord said. He moved over between Carrie and Jon. "Tell us where the money is and put a stop to all of this nonsense."

"We don't know where ..." Carrie started to say.

While still looking at Jon, Alvord sharply struck her in the temple with his elbow. Her head jolted to the side. She let out a clipped scream. He ignored her. Then he stepped around so that he could look directly into Jon's face. He moved closer, about a foot away. He brought his head down to Jon's eye level.

"This unpleasantness with Detective Able needn't have happened, you know." His voice was soft, almost soothing. "This whole thing is your fault, yours and hers." He nodded toward Carrie. "You could've prevented it if you'd wanted to." His eyes locked onto Jon's. "You have the power to stop it right now. All you have to do is …"

Jon answered with an ear shattering primal scream. He lurched his chair forward. He tried to smash his head into Alvord's face. Alvord jumped back on his heels and almost fell over. The scream continued. Jon twisted violently against his restraints. He crashed his chair over onto its side. His head smacked into the hardwood floor. Blood ran from his nose. He pulled and twisted inside the tape. It held fast. He strained to look over at Karen. The scream died away. Tears ran down his face. "Goddamn you, you bastards!" The tears wouldn't stop.

"My, my." Alvord regained his composure. He stood looking down at Jon on the floor.

"You watching this, doc?" Chestnut said to Carrie. "You taking it all in? I certainly hope so, because if nobody talks, once we've finished with her, we're starting on you."

"You bastards!" Jon spit out the words. He twisted his head up off the floor. His neck veins filled with blood and stood out from the side of his neck. His face was flushed a deep crimson. "You're not getting away with this. I'm not letting you get away with this." He began thrashing again. He twisted against his bindings. He stretched against the back of the chair. He pounded against the floor.

"Jon," Chestnut said. She watched him struggle for a moment.

He kept fighting against his bindings.

"Jon!" she said again. He slowed just a bit.

"Jon," she said a third time. "While you're beating yourself up down there, I want you to think about this." He bucked against his chair. Chestnut let him struggle for a moment more, and then she put her foot on the side of his neck. She stepped down; he choked out a cough. She slowly increased the pressure until he stopped bucking, and he choked again. "There, that's better." She released a little of the pressure. "Now take a breath. I want you to focus." She paused a moment. "My job here is to get you to focus." Then she moved her foot up onto Jon's face and twisted it into the side of his ear. Jon groaned, but he remained still. His struggling had stopped. He didn't move. "Now, are you focused?" His eyes suddenly dried. She waited and then nodded. "I think so.

"Come on, Chap." She lifted her foot. "Let's go into the other room and leave these people alone with their thoughts." Alvord and Chestnut started moving away. She glanced back over her shoulder at Jon as she walked. "We'll be back when she wakes up."

Jon glared back at her. His tears were totally gone now. They'd dried up. They'd been replaced by something else. Chestnut hadn't noticed, but his tears had been replaced by pure, scalding, unadulterated rage.

:　:　:

Jon slid around so that he could look toward the room behind them. The door was three-quarters open, and Chestnut stood somewhere near the entrance. He could see her shadow, but for the moment the door shielded him from view. Alvord was totally out of sight.

"Are you guys behaving yourselves?" Chestnut asked. "Or maybe planning your escape? Remember, I want you to focus, but take your time. We want Karen fully recovered before we start in again."

Carrie half-whispered, "What are we going to do?"

"I heard that," Chestnut said from the other room.

Jon didn't hear it. Chestnut had done her job well. He was truly fully focused. He closed his eyes. He gritted his teeth. He tensed his muscles. He stretched his legs down as far as they'd go. He arched his back. He strained. Beads of sweat popped out on his forehead. He pushed as hard as he could. He called on all of his reserves. He pushed with everything he had. The chair creaked ever so slightly. He kept up the tension. He wouldn't let up. Nothing could make him let up. The back of the chair loosened from the seat, an arm came off, and then it came apart at the joints. His arms were free. He ripped the tape away.

"What's going on in there?" It was Chestnut's voice again.

Jon knew that he didn't have much time. He started to move. He got up and stepped toward the door. He grabbed one of the heavy chair legs.

Chestnut pushed the door open. Jon cocked the chair leg behind him like a baseball bat, and then he swung. It hit Chestnut just as she turned to see what was going on. He caught her square in the face. Blood splattered everywhere. Teeth went flying. Bones crunched. Her head snapped back, and then she went down. It took a moment for Alvord to register what was happening.

Alvord's gun was in a holster on his belt. Jon burst into the room and was on him before Chestnut hit the floor. He swung his club at Alvord's head, but as he swung, he caught a glimpse, with his peripheral vision, of Sergeant Tindall lying in a corner.

His face was mottled, and he was lying in a pool of blood. The distraction gave Alvord just enough time. He turned away just as the chair leg swished by.

Alvord was a trained professional, and he had every advantage. He instantly calculated the momentum of Jon's move. He completed his turn, swung all the way around, and then hit Jon hard in the kidney. But Jon was filled with an unfeeling blind rage. He took the blow.

Alvord stepped back and pulled his gun. Jon swung again and this time connected with his right shoulder. The shoulder cracked. The gun went flying. Jon drew his club back, ready to strike again. Alvord spun in the opposite direction as he swung. He landed a spin kick on the side on Jon's head while Jon's club only glanced off his back.

Jon went down. He hit hard. Alvord aimed another kick. Jon rolled into it and swung his club. He connected with the side of Alvord's knee. His leg buckled inward. They struggled on the ground, rolling over each other, but now Jon had the advantage.

Alvord's right shoulder was injured, and his right arm was weak. Even so, he still managed to land an elbow in Jon's ribs and then to break away for the gun.

The gun was about seven feet away. Jon lunged into the air and swung his club. It hit Alvord's injured right shoulder. Alvord screamed. Jon pulled him back by his leg, all the way back, so that his head was in striking range. Then he got up on his knees. He swung once more, this time using both hands. He brought the club down with all the force he could muster. The back of Alvord's head cracked. His body spasmed; his left side shook for a few seconds. Then everything went limp.

:   :   :

"Jon!" It was a scream. Carrie was yelling from the other room. "Jon!"

Jon glanced over toward the door.

The doorframe was empty.

Chestnut was gone.

He dove for the gun.

:   :   :

"Jon, she's in here," Carrie screamed. "She's in here, and she's after something in her purse." She screamed again, "Jon, there's a gun!"

Jon crashed through the door. Chestnut was standing next to a small corner table against the wall to his right. Her face was a bloody mess, almost unrecognizable. Her purse was in her left hand. Her right hand was wrapped around a pistol grip, and the gun was partially out. She froze when she saw Jon, who had Alvord's Glock automatic out in front of him, pointing directly at her chest. He was about ten feet away.

Carrie yelled, "Shoot her!"

Jon hesitated.

Chestnut held her hands still. She looked into Jon's eyes. She held fast for a moment. She assessed. She thought she saw uncertainty. Her left eye twitched.

Jon pulled the trigger.

**Bang**!

The shot hit her in the shoulder and spun her around. She dropped her gun and braced herself against the wall. He fired again. The second shot missed wide to the right. He fired twice more, and both bullets struck, hitting her in the back. She slid down to the floor. He stepped forward to close the distance between them. He fired again. Her body lurched. And then he fired again, and again, and again.

"Jon!" It was Carrie. "Stop!"

Jon kept firing. He emptied the magazine. He pulled the trigger until the chamber jacked open. He continued pulling the trigger.

"Jon!" Jon looked away, then at Carrie. "Jon, stop it. Snap out of it! She's dead."

He dropped the gun and rushed over to Karen's side.

# Chapter 42

THE THURSDAY-AFTERNOON crowd in the Blue Moon Café was smaller than usual. It was the end of the month, Bobby Arnold was retiring, and it was his last day on the job. He'd been the head bartender there for as long as anyone could remember, and now David Lewis, his former assistant, was taking his place. DeDe, as he preferred to be called, had lost a bet. He was wearing his best dress for the occasion. Jon and Karen were sitting with Bobby in a back booth, reminiscing about old times.

"You want another Redhook?" Bobby asked.

"DeDe will get it. It's his job now." Jon held up his hand to get DeDe's attention.

"Make that two," Karen said. Bobby rarely drank, but today he was drinking gin. They were talking about the events in Ocean City.

"That last story you wrote about the Sisters of Mercy affair was the cat's meow; it was your best," Bobby said. "The others were good, but that last one had real punch. It was the best of the series." He took a sip of his martini. "You should be thinking Pulitzer."

"It would be his second," Karen said. "He's a hell of a writer."

"He's a hell of a shot, too," Bobby chuckled, "considering that he'd never touched a gun before in his life. How'd you know that the bullets come out of the pointy end?" Bobby snorted out a laugh. Forensic reports had revealed that only 50 percent of Jon's shots had hit his target. The other 50 percent had gone into the wall, and that was from an almost point-blank range.

"He did what he had to do," Karen said. She was resting her injured hand, propping her elbow on the table. It had been almost a month since her injury. The bones in her finger had been rebuilt with cadaver tissue from a tissue bank and then pinned and wired to a titanium traction device fastened to her wrist. If everything went well, the device would be removed after another two weeks. Then she'd be fitted for a simple splint.

"You know what I don't understand," Bobby said, "the audiovisual system in Wolfson's room. I don't buy the explanation Alex Morse gave you for your article. I don't care if it would save a bunch on nursing staff; it's too much of an invasion of privacy to be a prototype for any kind of a larger patient-monitoring system."

"Neither do I," Jon answered, "But that's her story, and she's sticking to it. Dr. Bolam, their chief of staff, backs her up. I've asked around as much as I could, and no one's come up with anything different."

Karen said, "Maybe she suspected who Stewart Wolf really was, and maybe she thought he might divulge something in his state of delirium. She certainly worked closely enough with him to possibly have figured it out. She could've been after the money, too."

"Well, we'll never know now," Jon answered. "There's no one left to contradict her."

Chap Alvord was dead. He'd died in the small Ocean City

bungalow. Ana Chestnut hadn't been so lucky. Although still alive, she'd never fully regained consciousness. Her existence was defined by the limits of a permanent vegetative state. It was the blow to her face that had done the damage, not the multiple gunshot wounds. She'd been kept alive by intravenous feedings, but now that an Oregon judge had ruled that the feedings could be stopped, it was only a matter of time before she died a Terry Schiavo death, death by dehydration. With no next of kin, the likelihood was that she'd either end up in the basement of the Sisters of Mercy Medical Center on a tissue-dissection table or in pieces out in the fields of the Pacific Northwest Forensics Laboratory. In either case it would be a fitting end to Jon's series of newspaper articles.

Carrie had finished her tour of duty in Ocean City and had graduated early from her residency program. She'd told everyone that she needed some time off and she needed to get away. She'd purchased an airline ticket for South America and had promised Jon that she'd send him a photo postcard of her posing in a bikini by the ocean at Ipanema. Jon had said that he'd watch for it, and when it finally came, he noticed that she not only looked stunning but that she also looked genuinely happy. It was the first time he'd ever seen her look that way.

DeDe brought Karen and Jon their replacement beers. Bobby asked for a replacement martini, and then he asked Jon and Karen if they had any exciting plans for the future.

"The future? Oh, I don't know," Jon answered.

"Probably the same old thing," Karen added.

"Geez, what's the matter with you guys? You're both lucky to be alive. You should take some time off, do something fun, get married, have a honeymoon. I've had several; they're great as long as you don't take them too seriously. Don't you know how short life is?" DeDe brought him his martini. Bobby complimented him on the service, said, "Nice dress," and then took a sip. He put his glass down and continued, "Now take your friend Carrie Williams; she knows how to live."

"Oh, I forgot to tell you guys," Jon said. "Carrie sent me this." He pulled the postcard of Carrie at Ipanema out of his wallet. "I got it in the mail the other day." He gave it to Karen. She looked it over and then passed it on to Bobby.

Bobby looked at the photo and whistled. "Wow! What a babe! She really knows how to fill up a bikini. Where was this taken?"

"Brazil," Jon answered. "She promised she'd send me a picture when she got there."

Bobby turned the card over. "There's nothing on the back, no note or anything."

"I know," Jon said. "There's no need; her smile says it all. In all the time that I knew her, I don't think I ever saw her smile."

"I'd like to make her smile," Bobby said with a little leer.

"Bobby?" Karen said. "Be careful now. There's a lady present."

Jon took a sip of his beer.

"I wonder whatever happened to the money." Bobby asked.

Karen shrugged her shoulders.

"We'll probably never know," Jon answered. "That little shit Frankie Wolfson took his secret with him to the grave."

"Well, he was a greedy son-of-a-bitch," Bobby said. "I don't know how anyone could do that, at least not on purpose, not with a clear conscience."

"You mean die with all that money hidden away and not tell anyone where it is?"

"Yeah, that's exactly what I mean. What a waste." He sipped his martini. "Money's meant to be spent, to be enjoyed. Somebody ought to get some use out of it."

"I don't think Wolfson ever much worried about his conscience," Karen said.

Jon took a slug of his beer and then another one. He finished it and then put his glass back down on the table. Karen waved at DeDe. He acknowledged her wave and drew another beer from the tap.

"Wolfson told Carrie about the stock certificates," Jon said. "And then he told her about the Bank of America safe deposit box and its key. Why would he have done all of that if he weren't trying to pass it on? We found the key with its engraved serial numbers, and the key fit the safe deposit lock. The only problem was that the box was empty."

Karen wrinkled her forehead. She took a sip of her beer. Bobby put his martini glass down. He looked at Karen and then shook his head. Jon looked at one and then the other. "What?" They didn't say anything. "What's the matter? What did I say?" Jon asked.

After a few more moments Bobby finally answered. "The key, the Bank of America key." He was still looking at Karen.

"Well, I'll be damned." She started to laugh. "No wonder Carrie had such a big smile on her face."

Jon looked puzzled. "What do you mean, the key? What about the key?"

Karen rolled her eyes. "It's the numbers," she explained, "the numbers engraved on the key. Bank of America safe deposit box keys are blank. They're always blank. It's standard bank practice; it's a part of their security system. If the key's ever lost, the person who finds it, or steals it, won't know what it's for."

"That's right," Bobby said. "That's the way they do it." He picked up his martini glass.

"How come I didn't know this?" Jon asked.

"Maybe because you never had anything worth locking up in the first place." He sipped his drink.

"Carrie did tell me that we were looking for numbers," Jon said. "We both went all over the box. Neither one of us gave the key a second thought. Could the numbers have been for some sort of offshore acount? Do you really think she figured it out?"

"Figured it out?" Bobby laughed. "She didn't have to figure it out; she already knew. Wolfson told her. She knew it all along. She scammed you!"

"No!" Jon glanced over at Karen.

"Come on, Jon," Bobby continued. "She got you to write her cover story. It's perfect. Now everyone in the world knows that the safe deposit box was empty. They all think the money was lost, and that includes the syndicate and the feds. I've got to hand it to her."

"Could she really have been that smart?" asked Karen. She sipped on her beer.

Bobby answered her question with a big grin over the top of his martini glass. DeDe delivered Jon's beer. Jon took a big swallow.

"Even if she did figure it out," Jon said, "she'd have had to take the numbers to wherever Wolfson stashed his stock certificates, and then she would've had to figure out how to retrieve them. It wouldn't have been all that easy. And then, of course, after she cashed them in, she'd have to hide the money. However many millions it was, it wouldn't be that easy to hide, not with both the government and the syndicate looking for it."

Jon picked up the postcard off the table and stared at the image of Carrie standing in the ocean. He shook his head. "A hundred forty-five! That's a good one."

"A hundred forty-five what?" asked Bobby. He swirled his martini in its glass.

"Million," Jon said. "A hundred forty-five million dollars. That's how much money Wolfson hid away."

They all sipped their drinks in silence for a few moments.

"Where do you think she is now?" Bobby finally asked.

Jon answered, "Someplace warm. Someplace where there's surf and a sandy beach. Someplace where she could take off that bikini and go swimming in the ocean." He was still looking at the postcard. "Someplace where no one would care."

Karen punched him in the shoulder. "Let's not get carried away with our mental imagery."

Bobby laughed and stood up. "I've got to go. DeDe's swamped over there. I think he needs an assistant." He watched DeDe work to keep up with his customers. "You guys can talk about this for as long as you want, but you're never going to know what really happened, not unless Carrie decides to show up someday and tell you all about it." He moved so that he could get a better look at the card over Jon's shoulder, and then he chuckled. "You know, I've got to hand it to her. She really does have a great smile."

# Acknowledgements

It is difficult to give all of the people associated with this effort the proper credit they deserve, but I will try. Many thanks to Colleen, Karen, and Sue Coffman for their input, to Ed Stackler for his patience and editorial expertise, and to Eileen Rosenthal and Julie Scott for their book and cover design. To Jon, Karen, John (whose real name is Jon), Carrie, Alex, Jim, Bobby, Ana, Karla, Nichole, and all the rest, thank you for your inspiration and tolerance.

A special thanks to Eve Alvord for her generous winning bid at an ARCS charity auction, winning the right to have her husband depicted in this story. Eve, I hope you enjoyed his character. I made him a bad guy and killed him just as you asked.

And throughout it all Vicki supported me just like she always does. It's nice to have one thing in life that you can always count on.

# Author's Note

*A Prescription to Kill* is a work of fiction, and the act of euthanasia depicted in its first chapter would have been clearly illegal under the current terms and conditions of Oregon's assisted-suicide law—and yet it happens every day of every year, more or less as I have described it, legally, in every state in the Union, including Oregon. Drugs are administered ostensibly for pain relief and sedation (usually morphine through an IV drip), but as an "unintended" side effect, heart rates are quieted, respirations are depressed, and lives are shortened through the euphemism of the "double effect" principle. This practice of assisted death with a proverbial wink and a nod to pain relief is deceptive and dishonest and is beyond the scope of any reasonable oversight. Those of us who practice or have practiced end-of-life medicine recognize that laws need to be changed.

The human-tissue-processing industry really is a largely unregulated billion-dollar business, and the uses of and charges for non-organ human body parts as described in this book are accurate. A human corpse really is worth about a quarter of a million dollars when cut up and dissected into parts.

Residents of Astoria, Oregon, will recognize a geographical

similarity between the location of the mythical Ocean City of this novel and their hometown. Names, locations, and myriad other details have been changed to protect the innocent, and sometimes the not-so-innocent.

Landmarks, institutions, and locations in Seattle have also been changed, primarily for my own amusement and for that of my friends. My apologies to the distinguished members of the Sunset Club.